Acclaim for the

"The ability to critically review the research is essential for optimizing patient care. This book provides a good introduction to this process and maintains a level of sophistication that is both helpful and reasonable for students, paraprofessionals, and other non-research-based disciplines. ★★★★"

—*Doody's Reviews*

"This book, written by leaders in our field, articulates and synthesizes evidenced-based practice (EBP) in a manner that is very accessible to the practicing clinician. For those clinicians in particular who have doubts about the whole concept, this book will be extremely valuable in forging a path to EBP that will be compatible with the vicissitudes of practice. Nothing else like it exists."

—David H. Barlow, PhD, Professor of Psychology and Psychiatry, Boston University

"An innovative pocket-sized primer written by three distinguished psychologists. . . . a handy how-to manual on using research evidence to guide clinical work. Together they present a pragmatic, step-by-step approach to accessing, interpreting and applying research evidence to one's own practice."

—*New England Psychologist*

"This is as fine a guide to the new world of evidence-based practice as any clinician could hope for. From formulating the question to finding the evidence, and from evaluating the research to applying it in practice, Norcross and colleagues have provided a much needed road map to the appropriate use of research data in clinical practice."

—Paul S. Appelbaum, MD, Professor of Psychiatry, Medicine and Law, Columbia University

"An excellent primer on most aspects of EBPs, including finding, evaluating, adopting, implementing and sustaining those innovations in routine practice. The guide is generally good at simplifying, cutting through complexity, and offering practical explanations that supersede the jargon that all too often infiltrates the field. The publishing of this book could not have come at a better time. The book includes a wealth of useful information about EBPs for both neophytes and experienced therapists."

—*PsycCRITIQUES*

Clinician's Guide to Evidence-Based Practices

Clinician's Guide to Evidence-Based Practices

Behavioral Health and Addictions

Second Edition

JOHN C. NORCROSS

THOMAS P. HOGAN

GERALD P. KOOCHER

LAUREN A. MAGGIO

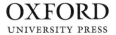
OXFORD
UNIVERSITY PRESS

OXFORD
UNIVERSITY PRESS

Oxford University Press is a department of the University of Oxford. It furthers the University's objective of excellence in research, scholarship, and education by publishing worldwide. Oxford is a registered trade mark of Oxford University Press in the UK and certain other countries.

Published in the United States of America by Oxford University Press
198 Madison Avenue, New York, NY 10016, United States of America.

Library of Congress Cataloging-in-Publication Data
Names: Norcross, John C., 1957– author. | Hogan, Thomas P., author. | Koocher, Gerald P., author. | Maggio, Lauren A., author.
Title: Clinician's guide to evidence-based practices : behavioral health and addictions / John C. Norcross, Thomas P. Hogan, Gerald P. Koocher, and Lauren A. Maggio.
Description: Second edition. | Oxford; New York : Oxford University Press, [2017] | Includes bibliographical references and index.
Identifiers: LCCN 2016027898 (print) | LCCN 2016028105 (ebook) | ISBN 9780190621933 (paperback) | ISBN 9780190621940 (ebook)
Subjects: LCSH: Evidence-based psychiatry—Handbooks, manuals, etc. | Mental illness—Treatment—Handbooks, manuals, etc. | Substance abuse—Treatment—Handbooks, manuals, etc. | BISAC: PSYCHOLOGY / Clinical Psychology.
Classification: LCC RC455.2.E94 N67 2017 (print) | LCC RC455.2.E94 (ebook) | DDC 616.89—dc23
LC record available at https://lccn.loc.gov/2016027898

Dedicated to
Veracious Evidence

Contents

About the Authors xi

Introduction xiii

ONE   Defining Evidence-Based Practice 1

TWO   Asking the Right Questions 17

THREE   Locating the Best Available Research:
Background and Filtered Sources 29

FOUR   Locating the Best Available Research:
Unfiltered Sources 49

FIVE   Reading and Interpreting the Research:
Research Designs 69

SIX   Reading and Interpreting the Research:
Numbers and Measures 109

SEVEN   Appraising Research Reports 137

EIGHT   Translating Research Into Practice 163

NINE   Integrating the Patient and
the Clinician With the Research 189

TEN   Incorporating Evaluation and Ethics 219

ELEVEN   Disseminating, Teaching, and Implementing
Evidence-Based Practices 247

Contents of the Companion Website 267

Glossary 269

References 285

Index 307

About the Authors

JOHN C. NORCROSS, PHD, ABPP, is distinguished professor of psychology at the University of Scranton, clinical professor at The Commonwealth Medical College, and a board-certified clinical psychologist. Author of more than 400 scholarly publications, Dr. Norcross has written or coedited 22 books. The most recent include *Psychotherapy Relationships That Work, Psychologists' Desk Reference, Self-Help That Works, Evidence-Based Practices in Mental Health: Debate and Dialogue, Insider's Guide to Graduate Programs in Clinical and Counseling Psychology*, the acclaimed self-help book *Changeology*, and *Systems of Psychotherapy: A Transtheoretical Analysis*, now in its eighth edition. He has served as president of the American Psychological Association (APA) Society of Clinical Psychology, the APA Division of Psychotherapy, and the Society for the Exploration of Psychotherapy Integration. Dr. Norcross has also served on the editorial boards of a dozen journals and on multiple professional committees, including the APA Presidential Task Force on Evidence-Based Practices. An engaging teacher and clinician, John has conducted workshops and lectures in 30 countries.

THOMAS P. HOGAN, PHD, is professor of psychology and Distinguished University Fellow at the University of Scranton, where he also served as dean of the graduate school and director of research, as well as interim provost/academic vice president. He served previously as associate vice chancellor for graduate and professional programs at the University of Wisconsin–Green Bay. Dr. Hogan has authored three textbooks—*Psychological Testing, Educational Assessment*, and *Bare-Bones R: A Brief Introductory Guide*—and coauthored several nationally standardized tests, including the Survey of School Attitudes and three editions of the Metropolitan Achievement Tests. He has authored numerous articles on measurement practices in such journals as *Educational and Psychological*

Measurement, Mathematical Thinking and Learning, and the *Journal of Educational Measurement,* and he is a regular contributor to the *Mental Measurements Yearbook.* Tom is a former member of the Exercise Development Advisory Committee for the National Assessment of Educational Progress (NAEP).

GERALD P. KOOCHER, PHD, ABPP, is professor of psychology and dean of the College of Science and Health at DePaul University in Chicago and editor of the journal *Ethics & Behavior.* He served as the 2006 president of the APA and, before that, as president of the Massachusetts and New England Psychological Associations as well as four APA divisions. Dr. Koocher formerly served as editor of the *Journal of Pediatric Psychology* and *The Clinical Psychologist.* He has authored or coauthored more than 250 articles and chapters in addition to 16 books. His text (with Patricia Keith-Spiegel) *Ethics in Psychology and the Mental Health Professions: Professional Standards and Cases* is the bestselling textbook in its field, and the *Psychologists' Desk Reference,* of which he is coeditor, is now in its third edition. Gerry holds specialty certification from the American Board of Professional Psychology in five specialty areas (clinical, child and adolescent, family, forensic, and health psychology).

LAUREN A. MAGGIO, PHD, is associate professor of medicine and associate director of graduate programs in health professions education at the Uniformed Health Services University, in Bethesda, Maryland. Previously, Dr. Maggio served as the director of research and instruction at the Stanford University School of Medicine, where she codirected the evidence-based practice (EBP) curriculum for medical students and provided EBP training for faculty and residents. Lauren has authored or coauthored more than 40 articles and chapters, including recent publications focused on best practices for teaching EBP.

Introduction

A warm welcome to the second edition of our *Clinician's Guide to Evidence-Based Practices: Behavioral Health and Addictions*.

We all recognize that clinical practice should be predicated on the best available research, integrated with the clinician's expertise within the context of the particular patient. Practice must be informed and guided by research. Yet so much of the research literature feels inaccessible and overwhelming, too removed and too large to guide what we do daily with our patients. Over the years, we also seem to have less time to retrieve the research, less capacity to understand new and complicated research designs, and, for some of us, fewer skills to electronically access the research.

We have designed this book to overcome these challenges to evidence-based practice (EBP); here, we provide you with the skills to retrieve and use research to benefit your patients suffering from behavioral and addictive disorders. Our book is a concise, practical guide designed to assist mental health and addictions practitioners in accessing, interpreting, and applying EBPs. It is a how-to manual on EBPs.

This *Clinician's Guide* features extensive text and multiple tables, like most books of its sort, but also case illustrations, clinical examples, skill exercises, glossary terms, and recommended readings and websites. In addition, the companion website on the Oxford University Press website features expanded content and interactive examples. Materials on that dedicated, free website are designated by 🖲 throughout the book. The website is: http://www.oup.com/us/cliniciansguide2e

The Audience

Our target audience is broad and multidisciplinary. We write for graduate trainees and busy practitioners in behavioral health and addictions who desire to access and apply the scientific research to more effectively serve their patients. Our audience includes psychologists, psychiatrists, social workers, counselors, behavior analysts, addiction specialists, marital and family therapists, and psychiatric nurses. It also embraces graduate students, interns, residents, and early-career clinicians of all theoretical persuasions. As emphasized in its subtitle, the book focuses on behavioral and addictive disorders.

Although EBPs rely heavily on the scientific research, we have written this guide for students and practitioners, not for researchers. We assume that readers will have completed an introductory statistics or research methods course and thus will have familiarity with measures of central tendency, correlation coefficients, control groups, and other foundational material. At the same time, most readers will probably require a refresher, which we provide, and will enjoy many reader-friendly graphics and helpful summaries, which we also offer throughout.

The Challenge

The goal of EBPs is to infuse clinical work with the best scientific research, thereby guiding practice and training. Doing so assures that our clients will routinely receive effective, research-supported treatments. Our students will receive training in those same treatments and will commit themselves to updating their competencies throughout their professional careers. In this respect, virtually every behavioral and addiction professional endorses the ethical and professional commitment to EBPs. Surely no one would advocate for the opposite: non-evidence-based practices.

While we enthusiastically support the goal of EBPs, we also harbor concerns about the reckless extrapolation of research from the lab to the consulting room and the insensitive imposition of premature EBP checklists onto clinicians and their clients. The clinician's contribution and the patient's voice form a crucial foundation for establishing a successful treatment plan. In this respect, we advocate throughout the book for inclusive EBPs that truly incorporate the three pillars of any EBP definition: best research evidence, clinical expertise, and patient characteristics.

The Content

The structure and contents of the *Clinician's Guide to Evidence-Based Practices: Behavioral Health and Addictions* reflect the delicate balance between research-guided practice, on the one hand, and clinician- and patient-informed practice, on the other. The optimal situation, of course, occurs when the extant research, clinician expertise, and patient values converge. However, we also address those situations where they do not.

In Chapter 1, we summarize the origins and definitions of EBPs. Several foundational controversies surrounding EBPs are briefly considered. We also introduce three clinically realistic and representative clients (Jonathon, Francesco, and Annique) whom we follow throughout the book to illustrate the real-life application of EBPs. From there, in Chapter 2, we focus on asking the right clinical questions—the beginning of any research-informed pursuit.

In Chapters 3 and 4, we outline the skills for locating the best available research: how to translate a clinical question into a targeted literature search, use search strategies, select search terms, access a wide range of information resources, and find information on tests and measures. The dividing line between the chapters is marked by the source of the research: background and unfiltered sources (Chapter 3) and filtered sources (Chapter 4).

Then a trio of interrelated chapters (5, 6, and 7) provides a practice-friendly refresher on research designs, numbers, and statistics and on the actual reports of research. Not to worry: We promise not to retraumatize any statistics-challenged practitioners. Instead, we remind you of the specialized vocabulary and appraisal skills you need to dip into the research literature in order to enhance your practice and, ideally, its effectiveness. We show particular concern about features of research designs and statistics that affect how you interpret results.

Once you are reacquainted with the fundamentals of reading and interpreting the research, we tackle in Chapters 8 and 9 the complexities of translating research into practice. Such translation cannot occur without carefully incorporating both patient and clinician into the process: the quintessential contribution of the behavioral health practitioner.

The closing two chapters address evaluation and education in EBPs. Chapter 10 demonstrates ways of evaluating the effectiveness and ethics of our clinical decision-making in EBPs. Chapter 11 features tips on disseminating, teaching, and implementing EBPs.

In short, the *Clinician's Guide* canvases the entire EBP process—asking the right questions, accessing the best available research, appraising the research, translating that research into practice, integrating that research with clinician expertise and patient characteristics, evaluating the entire enterprise, attending to the ethical considerations, and, when done, moving the EBP process forward by teaching it to others.

The Changes

In this second edition, we have thoroughly revised and updated the content; approximately a quarter of the material in the book is new. A host of other changes include

◆ a separate, focused chapter (3) on filtered sources for accessing the best available research;

◆ a new coauthor, Lauren Maggio, an evidence-based health librarian previously at the Stanford University School of Medicine and now at Uniformed Services University of the Health Sciences;

◆ a series of hands-on Skill Exercises in each chapter to provide practical use of the material, most of which should require only a few minutes to complete and all of which will help the material "sink in" (look for the boxed text designated by the symbol ☑);

◆ a new section on how behavioral health practitioners can optimally locate the desired research guidance, in contrast to how they actually search for it;

◆ a lengthier chapter (11) on dissemination and implementation to cover the burgeoning new field of implementation science;

◆ a reorientation of the chapters on evaluating research studies to focus more on reading and interpreting meta-analytic and Cochrane summaries and less on the designs of individual studies;

◆ a new section on barriers to successful implementation in the closing chapter;

◆ a slightly tweaked subtitle of the book—changing "mental health" to "behavioral health" to use the more contemporary and inclusive term;

◆ a companion website for the book at Oxford University Press (http://www.oup.com/us/cliniciansguide2e), with expanded content, interactive examples, and hyperlinked references (look for the boxed text designated by the symbol 🖥 for these additional EBP aids and resources); and

◆ a dozen online modules from the book's coauthors featuring EBP content and skill enhancements; these free, 15-minute mini-webinars take you beyond the text to practical examples and advanced discussions.

Despite these revisions and additions, our original mission endures: The *Clinician's Guide to Evidence-Based Practices: Behavioral Health and Addictions* remains a concise, practical, how-to book intended for graduate students and behavioral health practitioners. We hope you find it useful!

Clinician's Guide to Evidence-Based Practices

Defining Evidence-Based Practice

THIS CHAPTER SETS THE STAGE FOR THE BOOK BY SKETCHING A BRIEF history of **evidence-based practice (EBP),** explicating the definition and goal of EBP, outlining the controversies about EBP, introducing three composite patients who will reappear as examples throughout the book, and identifying the core skills in conducting EBP. As befits a how-to manual, we leave it to others (see Recommended Readings and Websites at the end of this chapter) to detail the history and debates surrounding EBPs in behavioral health and addictions.

Short History of Evidence-Based Practice

Evidence-based practice has a long past but a short history. The long past entails hundreds of years of effort to base clinical practice on the results of solid research. Starting with its separation from philosophy and Wilhelm Wundt's early laboratory experiments, psychology has always prided itself on having deep scientific roots. Similarly, from Emil Kraepelin's diagnostic scheme to Benjamin Rush's empirical efforts, psychiatry has also tried to establish itself as a science of mind (Norcross et al., 2006a). Addiction treatment, having its origins in Alcoholics Anonymous and self-help traditions, was slower to embrace empirical foundations but has increasingly been guided by scientific research.

The short history of EBP in behavioral/mental health traces back to the 1980s, originally in Great Britain and then gathering steam in Canada, the United States, and now around the globe. Many trace the early stirrings of the movement back to the United Kingdom and Archie Cochrane's (1979) article calling on medicine to assemble critical summaries of the scientific treatments that have proven effective according to randomized clinical trials. His seminal idea culminated in the Cochrane Collaboration (reviewed in Chapter 4), an exemplar of expert reviews of the research evidence. Cochrane and others contrasted evidence-based practice with expert- or **authority-based practice**, which lacks solid research support and typically results in less effective health care. The McMaster University Group in Canada (ebm.mcmaster.ca/) is frequently credited with refining the EBP process and focusing on the critical appraisal of the research evidence.

The EBP movement initially concerned medicine—**evidence-based medicine (EBM)**—but quickly spread to other health professions, such as nursing, dentistry, and physical therapy. In fact, EBPs came relatively late to behavioral health and the addictions. Thus, much of the vocabulary, for better and for worse, has come from the pioneering effort in EBM.

Since the early 1990s, we have witnessed impressive growth in the number of articles invoking EBPs. Figure 1.1 presents the annual number of citations for "evidence based" since 1992 in three national databases: MEDLINE (medicine), CINAHL (nursing and allied health care), and PsycINFO (psychology; also see Walker et al., 2006). Truly, EBP has become an international juggernaut.

In behavioral or mental health, the EBP movement has become most visible (and controversial) in identifying certain "evidence-based" treatments in the form of compilations, lists, and guidelines and then publicizing these to practitioners, training programs, and healthcare payers. The following are a few prominent examples:

◆ Task forces of several American Psychological Association (APA) divisions have published compilations of evidence-based or empirically supported treatments. These exist for children, adolescents, adults, and older adults suffering from a multitude of disorders. In addition, several APA divisions and other organizations

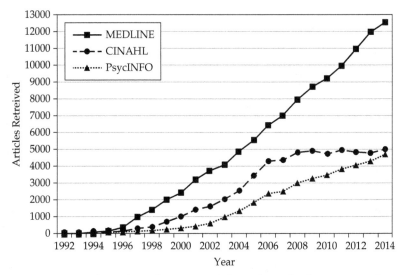

FIGURE 1.1 Number of articles retrieved from three databases using the search term "evidence based."

have enlarged the scope of EBPs beyond treatments to embrace evidence-based therapeutic relationships (Norcross, 2011), clinical assessments (Hunsley et al., 2004), and principles of change (Castonguay & Beutler, 2006). Evidence-based practice rightfully applies to all clinical services, not only treatment.

◆ The American Psychiatric Association has published 16 practice guidelines on mental disorders ranging from schizophrenia to anorexia to nicotine dependence. Although only recently identified as explicitly "evidence based," these and similar guidelines have identical intent: Use the best available knowledge to compile statements of "what works" or "best practices." Literally hundreds of healthcare guidelines are now widely available (see the National Guideline Clearinghouse at www.guideline.gov).

◆ The Substance Abuse and Mental Health Services Administration (SAMHSA) has created the National Registry of Evidence-Based Programs and Practices (www.nrepp.samhsa.gov), designed to provide the public with reliable information on the scientific value and practicality of interventions that prevent or treat behavioral and substance abuse disorders.

◆ State and federal governments have entered the evidence-based arena for virtually every health and social malady. Documents and websites appear almost daily on EBPs for such priorities as reducing healthcare disparities (e.g., the Health Care Innovations Exchange, www.innovations.ahrq.gov), preventing substance abuse (www.ncjrs.gov/ondcppubs/publications/prevent/evidence_ based_eng.html), and decreasing unwanted pregnancy (www.hhs. gov/ash/oah/oah-initiatives/teen_pregnancy/db/).

Evidence-based practices have profound implications for practice, training, and policy. What earns the privileged designation of "evidence based" will increasingly determine, in large part, what we practice, what we teach, and what research wins funding. In some jurisdictions, reimbursement for assessment and treatment services depends on their gaining designation as EBPs.

The long past but short history of EBP will increasingly require professionals to base their practice, to whatever extent possible, on research evidence. No profession can afford to sit on the sidelines; no practitioner can afford to ignore the juggernaut.

 The companion website to this book contains hyperlinks to policy statements on EBP by a number of professional associations, including the APA and many healthcare organizations.

Definition of Evidence-Based Practice

A consensual and concrete definition of EBP has emerged from the literature. Adapting a definition from Sackett and colleagues, the Institute of Medicine (IOM, 2001, p. 147) defined *evidence-based medicine* as "the integration of best research evidence with clinical expertise and patient values." The APA Presidential Task Force on Evidence-Based Practice (2006, p. 273), beginning from this foundation and expanding it to mental health, defined *evidence-based practice* as "the integration of the best available research with clinical expertise in the context of patient characteristics, culture, and preferences." We will use the latter as our operational definition throughout this book.

Several core features of EBPs become manifest in this definition. First, EBPs rest on three pillars: available research, clinician expertise, and patient characteristics, culture, and preferences. By definition, the wholesale imposition of research without attending to the clinician or patient is *not* EBP; conversely, the indiscriminate disregard of available research is *not* EBP.

Second, the definition requires integrating these three evidentiary sources. The integration flows seamlessly and uncontested when the three evidentiary sources agree; it becomes complicated and contested when the three sources disagree (see Chapters 8 and 9).

Third, the three pillars do not all stand equal: Research assumes priority in EBP. Clinicians begin with research and then integrate it with their expertise and patients' values.

Fourth, compared with EBM, the patient assumes a more active, prominent position in EBP in behavioral health and addictions. "Patient values" in EBM rise to the status of "patient characteristics, culture, and preferences" in behavioral health EBPs.

Fifth, the treating professional performs the integration and makes the final determinations in collaboration with the patient. The practitioner makes the ultimate judgment regarding a particular intervention or treatment plan. Treatment decisions should never rest in the hands of untrained people unfamiliar with the specifics of the case.

Sixth and final, EBP concerns using, *not* doing, research. Nothing in the EBP movement demands that practitioners conduct original research. Rather, the definition emphasizes that practitioners consume and translate the extant research into their routine clinical practice.

Part of the contention surrounding EBP revolves around the definitions of its three constituent pillars. Below we offer definitions of each pillar, borrowing from the APA Presidential Task Force (2006).

♦ **Best available research:** clinically relevant research, often from basic health science, that will most likely yield accurate, unbiased, and relevant answers to the practice question posed for a particular patient or patient group. The research can relate to prevalence, treatment, assessment, disorders, and patient populations in laboratory and field settings. Such research evidence should flow from a foundation of systematic reviews, reasonable effect sizes, statistical and clinical significance, and a body of supporting evidence.
♦ **Clinical expertise:** the clinician's skills and past experiences that promote positive therapeutic outcomes, including conducting assessments, developing diagnostic judgments, making clinical

decisions, implementing treatments, monitoring patient progress, using interpersonal expertise, understanding cultural differences, and seeking available resources (e.g., consultation, adjunctive or alternative services) as needed. Integral to clinical expertise is an awareness of the limits of one's skills and attention to the heuristics (biases) that can hamper clinical judgment.

♦ **Patient characteristics, culture, and preferences:** the personality, strengths, sociocultural context, unique concerns, and preferences that the patient (or patient group) brings to a clinical encounter and that must be integrated into clinical decisions to best serve the patient. Clinical decisions should evolve in collaboration with the patient and in consideration of the probable costs, benefits, and available resources. Individual patients may require unique decisions and interventions not directly addressed by the available research. The involvement of an active, informed patient will generally prove crucial to the success of mental health and addiction services. (We will occasionally use *patient characteristics* as an inclusive shorthand for the cumbersome *patient characteristics, culture, and preferences.*)

 Skill Exercise 1-1

Type "definition of evidence based practice" into your favorite browser and spend a few moments reading the results. How well do the definitions converge? How many of the website definitions specifically mention research as an evidentiary source? (Probably all of them.) How many definitions correctly identify all three pillars of EBP? (Probably only a few.) How many of them emphasize the roles of an active, informed patient and of culture? (Not many either.) This exercise will likely help you appreciate the inconsistency and misconceptions surrounding the definition of EBP.

Goal of Evidence-Based Practice

Here, we have perfect unanimity. The overarching goal of EBP lies in promoting effective behavioral health and addiction practices. As applied to individual clinicians, EBP should increase the efficacy, efficiency, and applicability of services provided to individual patients (or patient groups). These services will include assessment, case formulation, prevention, therapeutic relationship, treatment, and consultation. As applied to society as a whole, EBP should enhance public health.

The Evidence-Based Practice Controversies

As any behavioral health practitioner can readily attest, language has enormous power. Freud famously remarked that words were once magic: "Words and magic were in the beginning one and the same thing, and even today words retain much of their magical power." Words can diminish or privilege.

So it is with EBPs. At first blush, we find near universal agreement that we should use evidence as a guide in determining what works. It's like publicly prizing motherhood and apple pie. Can anyone seriously advocate the reverse: non-evidence-based practice?

If you desire to initiate a bar fight among behavioral health professionals, just spark it by saying "evidence-based practice." Some practitioners will vilify EBPs as simplistic cookbooks imposed by bean counters and academicians that ignore the reality of real-world practice and the centrality of the therapeutic relationship. Others will insist that EBPs constitute a core competence for health professionals in the 21st century, demonstrably enhance the effectiveness of services, and direct clinicians to better ways of practicing. All will agree that EBPs challenge old-time beliefs and some current practices.

But the dichotomy is neither as simple nor as consensual as that. Deciding what qualifies as evidence, applying research to individual cases, and determining the optimal balance of research, clinical expertise, and patient values are complicated matters with deep philosophical and huge practical consequences. While unanimity exists regarding the purpose of EBPs, the path to that goal is crammed with contention—what some have described as the "EBP culture wars" (Messer, 2004).

By way of review, here are 10 controversies concerning EBPs (see Norcross et al., 2006a, for point–counterpoint arguments on each controversy).

1. ***What qualifies as evidence of effective practice?*** Yes, all three pillars—best available research, clinical expertise, and patient characteristics. But which should assume priority? If clinician expertise based on personal beliefs and clinical experiences stands as an equal component of "evidence" unchecked against objective criteria, then clinical expertise may become a source of bias in judgment and the very source of error that controlled research was designed to overcome.

2. ***What qualifies as research for effective practice?*** The easy answer holds that we should employ different research methodologies to address different clinical questions: for example, epidemiological research to ascertain prevalence rates; process–outcome research to demonstrate specific clinician behaviors that produce favorable outcomes; effectiveness research to address whether a treatment works in naturalistic, real-world settings; and **randomized clinical trials (RCTs)** to determine treatment efficacy. But the harder answer depends on the degree to which we in mental health rely, as medicine does, on the "gold standard" of RCTs to determine "what works." A spirited debate centers on the privileged status accorded to RCTs and their placement at the zenith of the hierarchy of evidence. Should case studies, qualitative designs, controlled single-participant studies, and effectiveness studies also have roles in determining effective practice?

3. ***What treatment outcomes should establish EBPs?*** Medicine often has physical, measurable indices of treatment outcome, such as laboratory measurements and pathology reports. By contrast, behavioral health and addiction have few physical indices and must rely on patient self-reports, even when reliably measured on valid tests. For some outcomes, such as pain and quality of life, medicine and behavioral science struggle together to find valid and reliable assessments. Should we trust patient self-reports, which tend toward reactive responses reflecting only one perspective? Should we employ more objective behavioral indices, therapist judgment, and external/ societal decisions on "what works"?

4. ***Does manualization improve treatment outcomes?*** Outcome research requires that patients receive similar, if not identically standardized, interventions. In medication trials, this

standardization involves administering the same medication at the same dose or following a standard protocol. In behavioral health research, this standardization has frequently involved the use of treatment manuals and observation checks to ensure fidelity. In fact, manualization has become a prerequisite for inclusion in most compilations of EBPs. While treatment manuals indisputably prove helpful for training and research, the research on their value in improving treatment outcomes shows mixed or null results (Webb et al., 2010). Should such manuals be required in clinical practice?

5. ***Do research patients and clinical trials accurately represent real-world practice?*** Evidence-based practice seeks to identify the most effective treatments in research studies so that we can widely implement those same treatments in practice. However, research findings do not automatically or inevitably generalize. Many hitches occur in generalizing from the lab to the clinic, in translating science to service. Just how representative are the patients in clinical trials? Can we safely extrapolate the research findings to our practice and to our patients? The degree to which we can confidently generalize remains a source of fierce debate.

6. ***What should we seek to validate?*** What accounts for effective treatment? In biomedical research, it is traditionally the specific treatment method—the medication, the surgery, the discrete method applied to the patient—that is credited for successful outcomes. In behavioral health and addiction research, however, we often find diverse perspectives and conflicting results. Some researchers and practitioners argue that the treatment method forms the natural and inclusive target for research validation, while others argue that the person of the psychotherapist and the therapy relationship actually account for more of the success and thus should become our targets for research validation and EBPs. In those instances, evidence-based treatments would give way to evidence-based therapists and evidence-based relationships

7. ***What influences what is published as evidence?*** The production, dissemination, and interpretation of research are inherently human endeavors, subject to the foibles and

failings of human behavior. No purely "objective" or "unbiased" pursuit of truth exists. As behavioral health professionals, we know that a multiplicity of factors, some beyond our immediate awareness, influence human behavior; conducting research is no exception. Research results fall under the inevitable influence of the researcher's theoretical allegiance, funding sources, investigator bias, and conventional wisdom. How trustworthy can we deem such research?

8. ***Do treatments designated as EBPs produce outcomes superior to non-EBPs?*** By definition, treatments designated as evidence based or research supported outperform no treatment and placebo treatment. We can confidently state that EBPs are superior to no treatment and sham treatments; however, we cannot state that EBPs necessarily qualify as "best practices" or "treatments of choice" unless they outperform bona fide, structurally equivalent therapies. It remains unclear and controversial whether EBPs reliably perform better than practices not designated as evidence based.

9. ***How well do EBPs address patient diversity?*** Neither EBPs nor treatments as usual satisfactorily address all of the dimensions of human diversity encountered in behavioral health and addictions. The patient's race/ethnicity, gender, sexual orientation, religious inclination, socioeconomic level, and disability status interacting with outcome have largely gone unstudied to date. The ensuing contention is to what degree EBPs, validated primarily on studies with majority populations, qualify as "evidence based" for marginalized or minority clients.

10. ***Do efficacious laboratory-validated treatments readily transport to clinical practice?*** Surely, we lose something in transport from the lab to the consulting room. Efficacious laboratory-validated treatments can transport to other practice settings and situations but do not necessarily do so. The degree and predictability of transportability have become bones of contention.

Reading this top-10 list alone might lead one to conclude that rampant professional discord exists regarding EBPs. And it does. At the same time, an impressive consensus also exists on the definition and objective of EBP, and we have observed a nascent convergence on many of the contentious points just discussed. We remind readers that this process is the typical response to innovation in the professions and the normal path of science: Innovations beget conflict and engender further research. In the meantime, practitioners move forward to provide their patients—and society as a whole—with the most effective, evidence-based services at their disposal.

Alternatives to EBPs

The Institute of Medicine's Committee of Quality of Health Care (IOM, 2001) concluded that the disparity between the healthcare that patients could receive and the healthcare they do receive is more than a mere gap; it is a chasm. Likewise, the President's New Freedom Commission on Mental Health (2003) pointed to a chasm between what we should practice and what we actually provide. Both national committees identified shortcomings in the *underuse* of proven treatments, the *overuse* of treatments for which there is little evidentiary support, and the *misuse* of even those treatments found to be effective. These and similar clarion calls signaled for many practitioners the clear need for EBPs in behavioral health and addictions.

If not EBPs, then what? If we do not follow robust evidence in reaching clinical decisions, then what might prove the alternative? In a humorous but biting article, Isaacs and Fitzgerald (1999) sarcastically argued that several alternatives to EBM exist, each based on the clinician's *personality*. Here are a few of them, adapted to EBPs:

♦ *Eminence-based practice*: The more senior the colleague, the less importance placed on anything as mundane as evidence. Clinical experience, it seems, is worth any amount of evidence in making the same mistakes over and over.
♦ *Vehemence-based practice*: The substitution of vocal volume for evidence. Browbeat your timorous colleagues and downtrodden students.
♦ *Providence-based practice*: Instead of evidence, let the clinical decision rest in the hands of the Almighty. God would know best, after all.
♦ *Nervousness-based practice*: Fear of litigation provides a powerful stimulus to overassessment and overtreatment. When in doubt, just avoid lawsuits.

♦ *Confidence-based practice*: Exemplified by surgeons, this approach calls for manifesting bravado in all circumstances and deciding the case based on unjustifiable confidence.

The serious point: Many alternatives to EBPs represent antiscientific regressions into individual personality and clinical experience alone. In *Great Expectations*, Dickens has Mr. Jaggers advise Pip "to take nothing on its look; take everything on evidence. There's no better rule."

Of course, that's not to say that other methods of using and envisioning evidence in clinical decision-making are incorrect. **Practice-based evidence**, for a prominent example, values research equally but finds that controlled experiments frequently prove infeasible or untransferable to real-world practice (Barkham et al., 2010). Instead, messy practice is documented and measured just as it occurs, rarely with any control of how practice is delivered. This strategy does not permit causal conclusions ("Does X cause Y?") but does address a no-less-important question: "How does adding X to the mix alter the complex system of the patient before me?"

Many practitioners find this type of research more compatible with their practice patterns and more accessible and culturally sensitive to their clienteles. The practice-based evidence approach certainly respects research, but it does not treat the RCT as the gold standard or the holy grail of science. The external or ecological validity of the research becomes prized over its internal validity, real-world effectiveness over laboratory-controlled efficacy. Fortunately, clinicians need not choose between the two: Evidence-based practice and practice-based evidence are complementary, not contradictory, visions of using research evidence to improve care.

 Skill Exercise 1-2

Here's a fun and informative exercise: Watch *Viva La Evidence*. It's a catchy, four-minute musical video on evidence-based healthcare that parodies Coldplay's song "Viva La Vida." The video presents a bit about the history of evidence and then its key principles. Access it on YouTube (www.youtube.com/watch?v=QUWoQ8tXVUc) or another site.

Three Patients

Let us introduce three composite patients who will reappear as examples throughout this book. We created these hybrids of clinically realistic and representative clients from among those we have assessed and treated over the years. Clinicians will immediately recognize common features in these clients, complaints, and contexts.

Jonathon is an engaging and rambunctious 8-year-old White boy, "smart as a whip but a real handful" according to his mother. Jonathon's preschool and first-grade teachers both suspected that Jonathon suffers from attention-deficit/hyperactivity disorder (ADHD). He underwent evaluation in first grade by the school psychologist. Psychological testing, behavioral observations, and record review supported a diagnosis of ADHD (mixed type) and mild-to-moderate oppositional defiant disorder accompanied by family tensions. Jonathon is the second of three children, ranging in age from 3 to 10 years, born to working parents (with health insurance) who have frequently separated and reconciled. The local pediatrician treats Jonathon's asthma with albuterol and offered to prescribe a psychostimulant for the ADHD as well, but Jonathon's father firmly resists any psychotropic medication at this time. Both parents are genuinely concerned about Jonathon and willing to participate in a few family meetings. However, their demanding work schedules and marital conflicts prevent extensive outpatient treatment.

Francesco is a quiet, polite 30-year-old Hispanic man who presents at a low-income primary-healthcare center with diffuse and moderate anxiety (generalized anxiety disorder) due to work and relational concerns. His first marriage ended recently in a divorce, and his $12 per hour factory job seems in jeopardy because of layoffs and outsourcing. His job does not provide health insurance, and as a single working man Francesco does not qualify for any heavily discounted state- or federal-funded insurance. The primary-care physician saw him twice for 12-minute appointments and learned of Francesco's extensive history of alcohol dependence, including two inpatient rehabilitations. Francesco admitted his alcohol abuse but minimized its effects. The physician referred him to the clinic case manager for counseling and referral.

Annique is an emotional and insightful 61-year-old African American woman presenting for outpatient psychotherapy to a psychologist in private practice. She works full-time as a high school teacher, as does her husband of 35 years. They enjoy excellent insurance benefits and job security. Her chief complaint of chronic depression (major depressive disorder) dates back to her adolescence. Annique has successively tried a number of antidepressant medications, which "take the edge off," and sees a private psychiatrist every three months for medication management. This course of psychotherapy will constitute her third. Her family history includes many close relatives with unipolar and bipolar II mood disorders. Annique is reinitiating individual psychotherapy at this time because her assertion deficits (exceeding the diagnostic threshold for dependent personality disorder) and menopausal complaints (particularly hot flashes and irritability) detract from the quality of her life and relationships.

Core EBP Skills

How, specifically, would a practitioner go about assessing, conceptualizing, and treating patients like Jonathon, Francesco, and Annique in EBP? By mastering a set of sequential **core EBP skills** or following the mnemonic **AAA TIE** or **triple A TIE**. We take up each of these skills in the following chapters.

*A*sking a specific, clinical question (Chapter 2)
*A*ccessing the best available research (Chapters 3 and 4)
*A*ppraising that research evidence critically (Chapters 5–7)

*T*ranslating that research into practice with a particular patient (Chapter 8)
*I*ntegrating the clinician's expertise and the patient's characteristics, culture, and preferences with the research (Chapter 9)
*E*valuating the effectiveness of the entire process (Chapter 10).

Key Terms

AAA TIE
authority-based practice
best available research

clinical expertise
core EBP skills
evidence-based medicine (EBM)

evidence-based practice (EBP)
patient characteristics, culture,
  and preferences

practice-based evidence
randomized clinical trials (RCTs)

Recommended Readings and Websites

APA Presidential Task Force on Evidence-Based Practice. (2006). Evidence-based practice in psychology. *American Psychologist, 61*, 271–285.

Barkham, M., Hardy, G. E., & Mellor-Clark, J. (Eds.). (2010). *Developing and delivering practice-based evidence: A guide for the psychological therapies.* Chichester, UK: Wiley.

Evidence-Based Behavioral Practice, www.ebbp.org

Guyatt, G., Rennie, D., Meade, M. O., & Cook, D. J. (2008). *Users' guides to the medical literature: Essentials of evidence-based clinical practice* (2nd ed.). Chicago, IL: McGraw-Hill.

Miller, P. M., & Kavanagh, D. J. (Eds.). (2007). *Translation of addictions science into practice.* London, UK: Elsevier.

National Guideline Clearinghouse, www.guideline.gov

National Registry of Evidence-Based Programs and Practices, www.nrepp.samhsa.gov

Norcross, J. C., Beutler, L. E., & Levant, R. F. (Eds.). (2006). *Evidence-based practices in mental health: Debate and dialogue on the fundamental questions.* Washington, DC: American Psychological Association.

Straus, S. E., Richardson, W. S., Glasziou, P., & Haynes, R. B. (2010). *Evidence-based medicine: How to practice and teach EBM* (4th ed.). London, UK: Elsevier.

2

Asking the Right Questions

FORMULATING A SPECIFIC, ANSWERABLE QUESTION CONSTITUTES
the first core skill of evidence-based practice (EBP) and lies at the
heart of accessing the best available research. Not all clinical questions can be answered by the research, nor do all research projects
answer specific clinical questions. This chapter focuses on asking the
right questions.

Clinicians have an average of one to four questions for every
10 patients they care for. However, they either do not pursue or do
not find answers to half of their questions (Del Fiol et al., 2014).
Subsequent analyses show that clinicians could in fact answer most
unanswered questions through improved query formulation. Thus
this chapter also focuses on asking answerable questions.

Why Bother Formulating Specific Questions?

Our students and colleagues frequently complain that this first skill
feels tedious and unnecessary; they want to "jump right into" the
research literature to secure answers. After a few hours of frustration and incomplete searches, they begrudgingly return to us and
request assistance. You must form an answerable clinical question

before beginning a literature search; otherwise, you will probably incur frustration and waste time.

The authors of the venerable *Evidence-Based Medicine,* now in its fourth edition (Straus et al., 2010, p. 23), argue that beyond preventing frustration and saving time, using well-formulated questions helps us by

♦ increasing the probability of locating evidence that is directly relevant to our patients' needs;
♦ focusing on evidence that directly addresses our particular knowledge needs;
♦ directing us to high-yield search strategies (see Chapters 3 and 4);
♦ improving our communication with colleagues in discussing cases, sending referrals, and receiving new patients;
♦ suggesting the forms that useful answers might take; and
♦ enhancing our satisfaction with EBPs by virtue of having our questions answered and our knowledge augmented.

We believe—but have no controlled research to support our belief—that behavioral health and addictions practice leads to a greater number and complexity of clinical questions than medicine. Mental health practice entails many types of interventions, in multiple settings, for a wide variety of potential patients. Practitioners work in hospitals, outpatient clinics, day programs, independent practices, schools, military posts, public health programs, rehabilitation institutes, primary-care facilities, legal settings, prisons, counseling centers, and nursing homes. We assess, diagnose, prevent, treat, supervise, research, write, and consult. Our multiple activities and varied work settings provide all the more reason for formulating specific clinical questions that yield answers that directly address our knowledge needs as they relate to specific patients.

Questions That Research Cannot Answer

As we marvel at the glories of scientific research, we should simultaneously acknowledge the outer limits of its applicability. Empirical research can inform but can never answer some of life's fundamental questions: What constitutes the good life? How do I define quality of life for myself? What does it mean to be a good person? What ethical principles should guide my life?

Research can generate crucial information on the incidence, effectiveness, and consequences of our moral and philosophical positions. It can tell us about the incidence of, say, rational suicide, the effectiveness of sexual abstinence programs, and the consequences of gun control laws. But research cannot directly determine personal values.

A Good Question Is Like a Beautiful Painting

In posing specific clinical questions, visualize patients as you might visualize a beautiful painting or photograph (Walker et al., 2006). Questions will naturally arise in both foreground and background. Foreground questions concern the immediate and specific case, whereas background questions ask about the general situation or setting.

Take the cases of Jonathon, Francesco, and Annique (presented in Chapter 1). Ask yourself (or your students and colleagues), what specific pieces of knowledge would you like to have in order to render them effective care?

Background questions concern general knowledge about disorders, tests, treatments, and any other healthcare matter. They usually begin with the words *who, what, where, how, why,* and *is* or *are,* followed by a particular condition or situation (Walker et al., 2006). Representative background questions for our three patients include the following:

What effective psychological treatments exist for attention-deficit/hyperactivity disorder (ADHD, Jonathon)?

Why would parents oppose the use of stimulant medication that might help their kid (Jonathon)?

What is effective treatment for patients who minimize their substance dependence (Francesco)?

What causes dependent personality disorder (Annique)?

How does depression relate to dependent personality disorder (Annique)?

In each case, note that the background question specifies two components: a question root (with a verb) and a disorder, treatment, or other healthcare matter. Rewrite questions in this format before proceeding further (Straus et al., 2010). Ask the questions you want answered, but do so in a format answerable by sophisticated searches.

Foreground questions have greater specificity and, when formulated in searchable terms, possess five components: the patient, population, or problem of interest; the intervention (broadly defined to include prevention, assessments, and treatments); the comparison intervention; the outcomes of interest; and the type of question you want to ask (Schardt et al., 2007). The best foreground questions take the form of a searchable format known as **PICO**: the *p*atient, *i*ntervention, *c*omparison, and *o*utcome. Some people refer to this format as *PICOT*, adding the *t*ype of question (therapy, diagnosis, prognosis, etc.) they wish to answer.

Practitioners are interested in both background and foreground questions. The relative proportion of each seems dependent on familiarity and experience with the particular disorder or treatment. Often practitioners find that by asking and answering background questions they find themselves transitioning to foreground questions. In medicine, for example, beginning clinicians pose more background (general) questions than foreground (specific) questions, whereas more experienced clinicians ask more foreground than background questions (Straus et al., 2010). Novices want and need different information from what experts want; our knowledge needs depend on our experience with a particular disorder or condition. But none of us ever becomes so expert as not to be faced with background questions.

 Skill Exercise 2-1

Read the following scenario and jot down a list of background and foreground questions that come to mind: As you finish up a session with your 54-year-old female patient recently diagnosed with alcohol addiction, she asks about the efficacy of group therapy and Alcoholics Anonymous (AA) for her condition. She adds that she thinks her insurance may cover group therapy, but she wonders about its demonstrated effectiveness for alcoholism. Lastly, she asks if you know of any research on the benefit of adding AA to the individual therapy you are conducting with her.

PICO Format

Today, most people search electronic resources using **natural language**, which usually consists of long phrases (or even complete questions). Many popular websites, especially search engines like Google, accept such searches. As you begin to use more specialized interfaces, however, you will find that natural language searches will not always yield the desired results. When this happens, it becomes important to break searches down into the PICO components identifiable by all search systems. PICO is most relevant for foreground questions.

Table 2.1 features the salient questions to ask yourself for each of the PICO ingredients. In this book, as throughout most of healthcare, we use the term *patient* for *P* to refer to the child, adolescent, adult, older adult, couple, family, group, organization, community, or other

TABLE 2.1 Questions to Ask for PICO

	Ask yourself . . .	Information to possibly include in your question
P **Patient**	Who is your patient? What is the patient population of interest?	Your patient's primary complaint, sex, age, race, history, or preferences (any factors that will influence your search)
I **Intervention**	What do you plan to do for your patient?	Specifics of your planned assessment or treatment (any therapies you are considering)
C **Comparison**	What alternatives to the treatment exist? (Sometimes there is no comparison.)	The alternative treatments (if any)
O **Outcome**	What do you think will occur after applying the treatment? What does your patient hope will occur?	The desired or hypothesized outcomes

population receiving behavioral services. However, we recognize that in many situations there are important reasons for using such terms as *client, patient population, consumer,* or *person* in place of *patient* to describe the recipient of a service.

The optional *T* in PICOT will prove useful in determining the type of question you seek to answer. The most common types of clinical questions pertain to diagnosis and therapy, but we can ask about many more topics: etiology, prevalence, comorbidity, assessments, prevention, therapy relationship, relapse potential, and so forth. Determining the type of clinical question helps you anticipate the particular kinds of studies (e.g., randomized controlled trials, case–control studies) to look for while searching. Table 2.2 presents several question types that a clinician may encounter, with corresponding examples of the PICO components.

For example, Francesco, your 30-year-old patient with an extensive history of alcohol dependence, returns to your office. He feels further stressed by his job instability and admits to drinking more heavily. You wonder if research evidence indicates that another round of inpatient alcohol rehabilitation would provide enhanced effectiveness. This scenario raises a therapy question; therefore you would likely seek a randomized clinical (or controlled) trial (RCT) or a summary review of RCTs. On the other hand, if your concern rests principally with an etiology question—like "Does Francesco's job stress contribute to his alcohol abuse?"—then you may find a cohort study more interesting.

Here is another, full example of the PICO strategy. You meet with Jonathon, your 8-year-old patient with ADHD (mixed type) and mild-to-moderate oppositional defiant disorder (ODD) accompanied by family tensions. Concerned about Jonathon but mindful of their time, his parents ask about the effectiveness of family therapy and refer to an article that they found online. They turn to you for research evidence that family therapy will warrant the investment of time and effort. Your initial instinct may direct you toward diving into the literature, but you should first formulate a solid, specific question using PICO (see Table 2.3). It might take the form "For an 8-year-old with ADHD (mixed type), ODD, and family tension, would family therapy improve the ADHD and ODD conditions compared with individual therapy?"

TABLE 2.2 Question Types and Corresponding PICO Components for Formulating Clinical Questions

Question type	Patient	Intervention	Comparison	Outcome
Therapy	An 8-year-old male with ADHD, ODD, and family tensions	Family therapy	Individual therapy	Improvement in ADHD symptoms
Diagnosis	A 63-year-old Native American female with possible dementia	Mini-Mental State Examination	No comparison	Accuracy of making diagnosis of dementia
Prognosis	A 45-year-old White female with a 20-year history of bulimia	Cognitive–behavioral therapy	Interpersonal therapy	Improvement in bulimia
Harm	A 19-year-old African American male with polysubstance abuse, resistant to treatment	Involuntary hospitalization or civil commitment	No treatment	Substance abuse in 6 months
Cost–benefit	A 31-year-old pregnant Hispanic female who deteriorates when off her SSRI medication	Maintenance SSRI for depression	No medication	Potential costs to fetal development
Prevention	A 14-year-old White female at elevated risk for illicit drug use	School-based prevention	Social competence intervention	Long-term drug use outcome

Note: ADHD = attention-deficit/hyperactivity disorder; ODD = oppositional defiant disorder; SSRI = selective serotonin reuptake inhibitor. Adapted from Gambrill (2012).

TABLE 2.3 A Specific Clinical Question Formulated with PICO

P **Patient**	8-year-old male with ADHD (mixed type), ODD, and family tensions
I **Intervention**	Family therapy
C **Comparison**	Individual therapy
O **Outcome**	Improved ADHD, ODD, and family functioning

Note: ADHD = attention-deficit/hyperactivity disorder;
ODD = oppositional defiant disorder.

Not all clinical questions will contain all of the PICO components. In fact, only 37% of questions involve both intervention and outcome. The research reveals that the PICO format centers primarily on therapy questions and proves less suited for representing other types of information needs, such as questions about prognosis and etiology (Huang et al., 2006).

Using PICO may not always seem immediately relevant to a particular clinical question. If you find yourself struggling with creating a PICO question, take a step back and simply divide your question into meaningful key components. That will increase the specificity of your question and thus the probability of securing useful answers.

Our advice to increase the specificity of your questions via the PICO format in EBP is, happily, evidence based itself. Using PICO or PICOT increases the proportion of specific questions asked (e.g., Villanueva et al., 2001) and the level of precision in the answers retrieved (e.g., Schardt et al., 2007).

 Skill Exercise 2-2

Consider a recent puzzling question or gap in your knowledge about the evidence-based ways to proceed in your daily practice. It could focus on assessment, diagnosis, treatment, prevention, supervision, or practically any clinical service. Formulate this knowledge need as a

PICO question. Start by identifying its key components and assemble them to formulate your question.

P -

I -

C -

O -

Clinical question:

Asking Patients the Right Questions

A well-formulated, PICO-formatted question assumes that you have already acquired a fair amount of information about the particular patient. You will gather such information by conducting an assessment, making diagnoses, and identifying patient strengths. In addition, we urge you to ask patients (and their significant others) a series of questions that will enable you to narrow your searchable PICO inquiry and tailor it to your patient's goals of care. These questions include the following:

♦ What **preferences** do you have regarding potential treatments?
♦ Are there any types of services you find *unacceptable* at this time?
♦ Do you hold strong preferences for practitioners in terms of profession, gender, ethnicity, language, religion, or sexual orientation?
♦ Are there important language or cultural considerations that I should know about?
♦ What have you tried in the past that seemed helpful?
♦ What have you tried in the past that did not help?
♦ Do you have health insurance or other means to pay for services?
♦ What are your time constraints and work and home schedules?
♦ What family and social supports do you have?
♦ What other professionals help with your healthcare?
♦ As we collaborate on a treatment plan, what else should I know about you, your values, and your situation?

The best-laid plans and the most evidence-based treatments often go awry because practitioners simply do not acquire (or consider) information on the individuality of the patient and the singularity of the situation. None of this should imply, of course, that we should prematurely settle for a suboptimal treatment plan; simply remember that forewarned is forearmed. Ask early to avoid later surprises and disappointments.

Prioritizing Searchable Questions

In a typical day of practice, the curious clinician will wonder briefly about dozens of questions—prevalence and comorbidity of disorders, validity of assessment tools, effectiveness of treatments, appropriateness of therapeutic relationships, applicability to patient characteristics, probability of reoccurrence, relevance of ethical codes, and so forth. However, very few of us have the luxury to immediately conduct an electronic search on the run or during practice hours. Instead, we must temporarily shelve our questions and then prioritize them for those brief periods we have to search the literature.

Deciding which of your many questions to pursue requires judicious prioritizing. Try this sequence of filters to prioritize (Straus et al., 2010):

♦ the urgency of the question to your patient's well-being,
♦ the relevance of the question to your learning and knowledge needs,
♦ the feasibility of answering the question in the available time,
♦ the prevalence of the question in your practice, and
♦ the personal interest the question holds for you.

Urgent, relevant, feasible, prevalent, and personally interesting questions should get your precious time. A moment of reflection will usually allow you to select from the multitude.

To answer clinical questions, practitioners must systematically formulate answerable questions in an efficient manner. The next core EBP skill involves locating and accessing research-based answers. That is the topic of Chapters 3 and 4.

Key Terms

background questions
foreground questions
natural language

(patient) preferences
PICO

Recommended Readings and Websites

BMC Medical Informatics and Decision Making, bmcmedinformde-cismak.biomedcentral.com/

Evidence-Based Behavioral Practice, www.ebbp.org/

Formulating Answerable Clinical Questions, ktclearinghouse.ca/cebm/practise/formulate/

PICO tutorials at guides.mclibrary.duke.edu/ebm/pico (Duke University) and learntech.physiol.ox.ac.uk/cochrane_tutorial/cochlibdo e84.php (Oxford University).

Richardson, W. S., Wilson, M. C., Nishikawa, J., & Hayward, R. S. (1995). The well-built clinical question: A key to evidence-based decisions. *ACP Journal Club, 123*(3), A12–A13.

Straus, S. E., Richardson, W. S., Glasziou, P., & Haynes, R. B. (2010). *Evidence-based medicine: How to practice and teach EBM* (4th ed.). London, UK: Elsevier.

Types of Clinical Questions, guides.dml.georgetown.edu/ebm/ebm clinicalquestions

3

Locating the Best Available Research: Background and Filtered Sources

A FTER FORMULATING A CLINICAL QUESTION USING PICO, as explained in the previous chapter, it is time to search for evidence-based research answers. But *where* should you begin? Should you look for a Cochrane Review, search Google, call a colleague, or consult a textbook? All of these are viable search options, but you will probably make better progress by beginning with a sound search strategy.

Librarians and experienced searchers recommend a definite sequence to the search process. Begin by searching background information, which provides an overview of your topic; then move on to filtered information (which we will define shortly), which provides access to timesaving synthesized information; and finally, if necessary, look into unfiltered information (addressed in Chapter 4), which provides access to primary sources, such as individual studies.

For example, say you begin a search on a professional organization's website (background information). After familiarizing yourself with the topic's main concepts and keywords there, you search the Cochrane Database of Systematic Reviews (a filtered resource).

Then, after consulting related Cochrane Reviews, you track down a promising original study in PubMed or PsycINFO (an unfiltered resource), which you then critique and apply.

Ideal Versus Typical Search Process

Ample evidence reveals a disconnect between this ideal search process and the typical search process of behavioral health practitioners. Most clinical psychologists, for instance, know of and occasionally access APA's PsycINFO or PubMed (Berke et al., 2011). These huge, unfiltered information sources easily overwhelm just about everyone. Trying to locate a consensus on best available research through these behemoths can feel like trying to find the proverbial needle in a haystack. Busy professionals need more accessible and relevant outlets that summarize the research findings.

Fortunately, that's what **filtered information sources** do: They distill decades of research evidence into practical, searchable resources. But few clinicians know about or routinely search these resources (Berke et al., 2011). Even doctoral-level psychologists, probably the behavioral health professionals most educated in statistics and research methods, do not access filtered resources frequently.

Thus in this chapter we present essential background and filtered information sources with a few introductory words on each. In Chapter 4, we cover sources of unfiltered information you can turn to should the filtered resources not address your questions or should you need to delve into the primary research itself.

Background Information

Background information sources provide a general understanding of a topic and sometimes also an overview of the available evidence. Unsurprisingly, background information is the most appropriate source for answering background questions (e.g., what side effects does this antidepressant have?). Background information appears in textbooks, topic review services like UpToDate, websites, and practice guidelines (all covered later in this chapter). At first, consulting background information may seem inefficient, but in the long run it can prevent frustrating and time-consuming false starts due to a searcher's lack of familiarity with a topic.

Background information can help a searcher identify a topic's specialized vocabulary or key researchers, both of which can be integrated into a subsequent filtered information search. A quick background search can also provide a sense of a topic's scope in the literature. For example, if you have difficulty finding background information on your topic, it may indicate that there will be even less filtered information available. In that case, you know that it may prove necessary to broaden your search as you move through the process.

Filtered Information

Filtered information sources are designed to save busy practitioners time and effort by providing expert analysis, thereby removing the burden of reading and synthesizing hundreds, or even thousands, of individual studies. Another benefit of filtered information sources is that in many cases they pull together a wide range of evidence that would otherwise be difficult to locate in one convenient resource. Filtered information sources include systematic reviews, meta-analyses, and enhanced critical abstracts.

The major downside of filtered information sources is that few of them exist, owing to the fact that filtered information takes longer than unfiltered information to create. This also means that it is difficult to find filtered information on current topics or rare conditions. Despite this drawback, we describe mostly filtered information sources in this chapter, because these are the most practical resources for most practitioners.

Remember: "Best available research" in EBP represents a research consensus of sorts across multiple studies conducted by independent scholars through many years. Think of results of meta-analyses or conclusions from systematic reviews, not individual studies. No single study, no matter how large or impressive, constitutes best available research. Filtered information provides the ideal way to access best available research to inform EBP.

Now that you have a general understanding of background and filtered information resources, learning how to best use them becomes critical. Fortunately, these information sources all usually operate with the same basic search concepts, so a strong grasp of the following search basics will make approaching any information resource less frustrating and less time-consuming.

Basic Search Concepts

Boolean Operators

Boolean operators are search commands used to logically connect search terms. The most common Boolean operators are AND and OR, although some search systems also allow for the use of the less common Boolean operator NOT.

AND narrows a search, making it more precise. For example, "depression AND alcoholism" retrieves information about both depression and alcoholism. A search using AND ensures that all retrieved citations contain information about both search terms. Figure 3.1 portrays the logical relationship of AND in the form of a Venn diagram.

By contrast, the Boolean operator OR broadens a search, making it more comprehensive. For example, "depression OR alcoholism" retrieves information about either depression or alcoholism. Figure 3.2 presents a Venn diagram of the conceptual relationship of OR.

OR can be helpful for stringing together synonyms. For example, to locate research information on depression, it would also prove useful to search for synonyms such as "mood disorders," "dysthymia," and "affective disorders." Therefore if you seek inclusivity, search for "depression OR mood disorders OR dysthymia."

The Boolean operator NOT negates or excludes information from a search. To continue with our example, "depression NOT alcoholism" retrieves only information about depression that excludes information about alcoholism. Use caution when applying NOT, as it can exclude potentially valuable information relevant to both

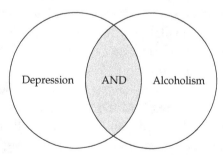

FIGURE 3.1 Venn diagram of the conceptual relationship of AND in electronic searches.

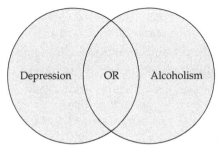

FIGURE 3.2 Venn diagram of the conceptual relationship of OR in electronic searches.

concepts. For example, the search for "depression NOT alcoholism" could omit a relevant article in which depression is the major focus and alcoholism a minor topic.

Boolean tips:

♦ Notation of Boolean operators can take different forms. For example, some databases may use "&" to represent AND. Take care to check each information resource's search tips.
♦ Boolean operators sometimes require capitalization to be recognized. Always capitalize Boolean operators, thereby ensuring compatibility with any databases that may require capitalization; those that do not will remain unaffected. Using capitalization also enables you to quickly see the logic of your search.
♦ Some search systems automatically insert Boolean operators between search terms. For example, Google automatically inserts AND between two or more search terms.
♦ Boolean operators can generally be used together in a single search thanks to a technique called "nesting." Nesting is generally notated by parentheses, for example, "(depression OR alcoholism) AND obesity." As in algebra, the parentheses command the search system to first isolate and search for the information inside the parentheses, then combine it with the search command outside the parentheses.

Wild Cards and Truncation

Wild cards broaden searches by automatically searching for variations on search terms. Wild cards, sometimes notated by the characters *, ?, $, or !, prompt the search system to identify possible alternate letters. In some cases, a wild card may retrieve a string of letters; in others, it may only substitute in a single letter. Wild cards can generally apply to any part of the search term.

Here are three examples of wild cards:

♦ "Practi!e" retrieves "practice" and "practise."
♦ "P$diatrics" retrieves "pediatrics" and "paediatrics."
♦ "Narcolep?" retrieves "narcolepsy," "narcoleptic," and "narcoleptics."

The last example above is also known as **truncation**. Truncation adds variations to the ends of search terms and can prove helpful when searching for plural forms of search terms. Some sophisticated search systems now search automatically for plurals.

 Skill Exercise 3-1

Based on a patient in your practice, you formulate the following PICO question: "For a 22-year-old female patient who did not respond to the maximum dose of an antidepressant, will augmentation with psychotherapy improve depression?" Describe the search string you would use to look for an answer to this question. Don't forget to include Boolean operators and, if appropriate, truncation or wild card commands.

Background Information Resources

We now return in more detail to background and filtered information, presenting the sources for each that are in common use among behavioral health and addictions practitioners. They are meant to be illustrative, not exhaustive.

The most common background information sources in this category are textbooks (including e-texts), eMedicine, websites, and practice guidelines. We consider each briefly in turn.

Textbooks

Textbooks are a common source of background information. In their print form, however, they tend toward obsolescence rather quickly, gradually losing their value as evidence resources. To combat this problem, publishers increasingly insist on frequent revisions and create e-texts, which can be updated more rapidly. In some cases, e-texts are simply online versions of traditional textbooks; in other cases, publishers create new, value-added online evidence components. For example, *Goodman and Gilman's The Pharmacological Basis of Therapeutics* (Knollmann, 2011), which has always been available in print, is now also available electronically by subscription through McGraw-Hill's Access Medicine collection at www.accessmedicine. com/. As an e-text, this title undergoes frequent updates based on emerging evidence, and the new references are also directly linked to the full PubMed citation, providing instantaneous access to primary evidence and ultimately saving a practitioner time and effort.

E-texts, available both online and for e-readers, vary in quality. Not all e-texts automatically update or include evidence features. Many libraries now purchase e-text subscriptions only, and you may want to investigate options for access to e-texts through your library. However, the National Library of Medicine does offer a free collection of e-texts that cover a variety of topics (www.ncbi.nlm.nih.gov/ entrez/query.fcgi?db=Books).

Hundreds of textbooks in behavioral health and addictions characterize themselves as "evidence based" these days. Some authors employ the term largely for advertising purposes, but others take the "the integration of the best available research with clinical expertise in the context of patient characteristics, culture, and preferences" as their primary intent. The latter category includes our favorite series of clinical texts from Oxford University Press—*A Guide to Treatments That Work* (Nathan & Gorman, 2015), *Psychotherapy Relationships That Work* (Norcross, 2011), *A Guide to Assessments That Work* (Hunsley & Mash, 2008), *Principles of Therapeutic Change that Work* (Castonguay & Beutler, 2005), and *Self-Help That Works* (Norcross et al., 2013)—and a series of brief books on particular disorders in the *Advances in Psychotherapy: Evidence-Based Practice* series published by Hogrefe. Even these dozens of texts, addressing both transdiagnostic practices and diagnostic conditions, cannot cover the entire waterfront of behavioral health and addictions.

As well, Oxford University Press publishes a series of paperbacks entitled *Treatments That Work*. Designed for practitioners and their clients, these books focus on communicating to busy practitioners evidence-based treatments and how they can implement them in their practices using step-by-step approaches. The series currently features approximately 100 titles; most are explicit guides for therapists and companion workbooks for clients. Each one focuses on a particular mental or addictive disorder. Books are for individual sale and also available on Oxford Clinical Psychology (www.oxfordclinicalpsych.com).

UpToDate

UpToDate (www.uptodate.com) is a topic overview resource promoted as offering evidence-based decision support for point-of-care use. It contains over 10,500 reviews of topics from 23 specialties, including psychiatry. Topics tie directly to current evidence when possible and then link directly to related PubMed citations, allowing for immediate access to primary evidence. UpToDate requires a subscription.

eMedicine

A continually updated evidence-based resource, **eMedicine** provides background information for over 30 medical specialties, including psychiatry, and has modules relating to addictions. Now a component of the broader information resource Medscape, eMedicine consists of the work of approximately 10,000 healthcare professionals, who have written or reviewed articles on over 10,000 diseases, drugs, and procedures. This resource's articles are dense but easily navigable, providing "practice essentials" that introduce the condition and then progressing into more detail regarding potential therapies (including specific information on drug therapy), prognosis, and differential diagnosis. Hyperlinked references abound throughout, allowing users to immediately link, when possible, to the complete PubMed citation for the reference. One can access all Medscape content online and via all major mobile devices.

A product of the company WebMD, eMedicine is available free of charge at emedicine.medscape.com/. Although free, the site does encourage users to register to personalize content based on their specialties. Readers will encounter a push toward trying WebMD's continuing-education products, and clearly marked advertisements appear on the majority of pages.

 The companion website for this book presents color screenshots of the websites of all the background and filtered information sources featured in this chapter.

Websites

As EBP continues to raise its profile in healthcare, its presence on the Internet increases. For example, many professional and government organizations have constructed EBP sites and regularly add research-supported information to existing websites. The Internet's instantaneous nature and flexible publishing policies also allow for the immediate appearance of research that is in press or that might never appear in print.

In relation to Francesco, your patient with an extensive history of alcohol dependence, we recommend beginning the search process at the Substance Abuse and Mental Health Services Administration (SAMHSA; www.samhsa.gov) website. This US government website features extensive statistical data at the national and state levels, descriptions of and links to training programs, and a wide variety of valuable reports, including reports from the Surgeon General. It might also refer you to the Addiction Technology Transfer Center Network (nattc.org/home), which SAMHSA funds. The SAMHSA site also provides access to a range of mobile apps for clinicians and consumers.

Importantly, SAMHSA features the **National Registry of Evidence-Based Programs and Practices (NREPP)**, a database of behavioral health and substance abuse treatments. Available at www.nrepp.samhsa.gov, this free full-text database provides intervention summaries, which describe each intervention and its targeted outcomes, comment on the research on the intervention, provide references for the intervention, and identify the individuals who developed the intervention. Ratings of evidence class and outcomes appear for each intervention, based on rigor, effect size, program fidelity, and conceptual framework.

Currently, NREPP contains over 380 treatments and preventive interventions, which one can quickly browse by clicking "view all." The database features a user-friendly search platform that allows searching by keyword, with the option of limiting searches to specific program types (e.g., treatments or preventions), geographic locations, outcome categories, or population groups. NREPP also includes a learning center, which supports clinicians in selecting, implementing, and evaluating EBPs.

 Skill Exercise 3-2

Spend a few moments getting acquainted with NREPP and its contents. Select a favorite disorder or treatment, and examine the entries. Like every EBP information source, NREPP has its strengths and weaknesses. We have identified many of its advantages above, but as a discerning practitioner, identify several weaknesses. You will find that among these are a dearth of assessment methods, an overreliance on manualized methods, a paucity of international contributions, and prizing new, branded therapies at the expense of established common factors. Even the terminology—"interventions"—irks some clinicians committed to more relational therapies. Although we respect NREPP, this exercise should attune you to the reality that no single information source will ever satisfy all clinical needs and theoretical perspectives.

Practitioners seeking research evidence on particular psychological treatments may also find discipline-specific websites of value. For example, the Society of Clinical Psychology (APA Division 12) sponsors a website focused on research-supported treatments for adult disorders (www.div12.org/psychological-treatments/). Similarly, several APA divisions provide access to a website focused on effective therapies for children and adolescents (effectivechildtherapy. org/content/more-about-specific-treatments). For trauma, the National Child Traumatic Stress Network manages a website that describes empirically supported treatments and promising practices for children (www.nctsn.org/resources/topics/treatments-that-work/ promising-practices). Note that these discipline-specific websites feature only psychological therapies (not other clinical services) for specific diagnoses.

No section on websites would be complete without a word on Google (www.google.com/). Google, the most popular Internet search engine, is a great resource; for many of us it has become the first place we look for information on just about anything. However, when using Google for behavioral health and addiction information, you may find it helpful to limit the search to only those websites in a specific domain. By using a certain command or the Advanced Search option, you can, for example, limit your search to just government (.gov), nonprofit (.org), or educational (.edu) websites, weeding out commercial (.com) sites.

Using the Google Advanced Search feature (www.google.com/ advanced_search), look for the "site or domain" search option and enter the domain range you seek. Or, if want to use the standard Google search box, simply input your search terms and the word *site* followed by a colon and then your specified domain range, e.g., *.gov*, *.com*, or *.org*. If seeking noncommercial sites on bipolar disorder, for example, you would enter "bipolar disorder site:.org" (note that there must be no space after the colon). This search will retrieve only sites on bipolar disorder ending in *.org*. You could also search for sites with *.edu* and *.gov* domains. Another specialized Google search feature, Google Scholar, will be discussed in Chapter 4.

Lastly, a Google search term commonly returns results from Wikipedia, the popular Web-based encyclopedia that provides background information in over 35 million articles on wide range of topics. Wikipedia articles can be created and edited by anyone with an Internet connection and generally include links to primary literature. There is great debate about the quality control of Wikipedia pages (Reavley et al., 2012). A recent review of 110 studies demonstrated mixed results for the content accuracy of its entries, although the positive evaluations of Wikipedia were more numerous than the negative ones (Mesgari et al. 2015).

Therefore if you are reading a Wikipedia article, we encourage you to check the article's references and "talk page." Wikipedia talk pages are a communication channel for editors to discuss edits of articles. Talk pages provide a sense of how the article was created and can help you make an informed decision about the trustworthiness of the information. Wikipedia bills itself as a starting point for research; however, if you would like to exclude Wikipedia articles from your Google search, simply use the character "-" to represent "minus" (e.g., "depression -site:Wikipedia.org").

As with any source, when using information from the Internet, act as a cautious and critical consumer. Keep the following questions in mind when using the Internet as a source of healthcare information:

- ◆ When was the site last updated? How current is the information?
- ◆ Who claims responsibility for the site? Is it a pharmaceutical company? A government agency? An academic institution?
- ◆ What is the motive behind the site? Is it asking you to purchase products or services?
- ◆ Does the site feature any references to scholarly sources?
- ◆ Do you trust the information on this site? Follow your instincts: If the information does not feel right, move on. There will be plenty of good, reputable information elsewhere.

 Skill Exercise 3-3

Search Wikipedia for a topic of clinical interest and on which you possess considerable expertise. Read its contents. Also review the entry's references, talk page, and history tab. Would you characterize the content as accurate, timely, and balanced? Are there any red flags? Are there any elements that surprise you? Consider how you may or may not want to use Wikipedia for background information.

Practice Guidelines

Practice guidelines, another valuable source of background information, have been defined as "user-friendly statements that bring together the best external evidence and other knowledge necessary for decision-making about a specific health problem" (Sackett et al., 1997, p. 112). In addition to providing background information, many guidelines increasingly provide direct links to current evidence.

Many guidelines appear on professional association websites or through clearinghouse sites such as the National Guideline Clearinghouse (www.guideline.gov) and the UK-based National Institute for Health and Clinical Excellence (NICE; www.nice.org.uk/guidance). Both of those sites are searchable and provide access to the full texts of EBP guidelines. For behavioral health and addictions, for example, the National Guideline Clearinghouse features over 450 specific mental health guidelines from relevant professional organizations, such as the American Academy of Child and Adolescent Psychiatry and SAMHSA.

For a list of background information resources, please see Box 3.1.

Box 3.1 Featured Background Information Resources

- ◆ Textbooks and e-texts
  - *Goodman and Gilman's The Pharmacological Basis of Therapeutics*: www.accessmedicine.com
  - National Library of Medicine's free e-texts: www.ncbi.nlm.nih.gov/entrez/query.fcgi?db=Books
  - Oxford Clinical Psychology and *Treatments That Work*: www.oxfordclinicalpsych.com
- ◆ UpToDate: www.uptodate.com
- ◆ Websites
  - Substance Abuse and Mental Health Services Association (SAMHSA): www.samhsa.gov
  - National Registry of Evidence-Based Programs and Practices (NREPP): www.nrepp.samhsa.gov
  - Discipline-specific websites on psychological therapies: www.div12.org/psychological-treatments/, effectivechildtherapy.org/content/more-about-specific-treatments, and www.nctsn.org/resources/topics/treatments-that-work/promising-practices
- ◆ Google: www.google.com
- ◆ Wikipedia: www.wikipedia.org
- ◆ Practice Guidelines
  - National Guideline Clearinghouse: www.guideline.gov
  - National Institute for Health and Clinical Excellence (NICE): www.nice.org.uk

---

Filtered Information Resources

Here, we consider several of the most frequently used and, in our opinion, the most helpful filtered information resources for behavioral health and addiction professionals:

- Cochrane Database of Systematic Reviews (www.cochranelibrary. com/),
- Campbell Collaboration reviews (www.campbellcollaboration. org/lib/).
- Database of Abstracts of Reviews of Effects (www.crd.york.ac.uk/ crdweb),
- *BMJ Clinical Evidence* (www.clinicalevidence.com), and
- evidence-based journals.

Cochrane Database of Systematic Reviews

The **Cochrane Database of Systematic Reviews (CDSR)** is a database within the Cochrane Library comprising over 6,000 systematic reviews that identify and expertly synthesize available randomized clinical trials (RCTs) on a given healthcare topic. Considered a "gold standard" of EBP in behavioral health, the CDSR is a great place to start searching filtered information. The CDSR is especially useful when searching for therapy information and less helpful when searching for answers to other types of clinical questions (although it includes some diagnosis-focused reviews). When searching the CDSR, remember that its reviews are time-consuming to produce, so if a topic is fairly new, it may not yet be covered. Also, because Cochrane Reviews synthesize related RCTs, a substantial number of RCTs must exist before a review can be undertaken. This makes the Cochrane a solid resource for established topics that have been thoroughly investigated in the healthcare literature, but it may prove hit or miss when it comes to new or rare topics.

The CDSR was created and is maintained by volunteer healthcare practitioners, biomedical researchers, expert searchers, and consumers who make up the Cochrane Collaboration, an international nonprofit organization. The CDSR is updated monthly; Cochrane encourages its reviewers to update their specific reviews at least once every two years. Despite best efforts, however, the suggested two-year time frequently gets extended.

Cochrane Reviews are dense documents but are divided into user-friendly sections. Reviews may include the following sections: implications for practice and research, author's conclusions, and descriptions and an analysis of the RCTs examined. Access to the full text of the CDSR online requires a subscription. Abstracts and plain-language summaries of Cochrane Reviews, which contain substantial and conclusive information, can also be accessed free through the Cochrane Library at www.cochranelibrary.com/ and PubMed.

Although the CDSR is available via several access points, we focus on the Cochrane Library site presented by Wiley (onlinelibrary. wiley.com/cochranelibrary/search/). This interface simultaneously searches the entire Cochrane Library, which also includes other EBP resources, as discussed later in this chapter and in Chapter 4.

Consider our question of whether family therapy or individual therapy has the stronger research evidence for being useful in treating Jonathon, our 8-year-old patient with ADHD, ODD, and family conflicts. In this case, ADHD, ODD, family conflict, family therapy, and individual therapy are the main concepts. In beginning our search, we choose "ADHD" because of its prevalence in the healthcare literature, and "family therapy" becomes the main therapy. A viable search string could look like 'ADHD "family therapy."' Inserting AND is unnecessary, because the Wiley interface automatically inserts AND between terms. We place "family therapy" in quotes to alert the database to search it as a phrase.

This relatively simple search yielded two highly relevant Cochrane Reviews: "Family Therapy for Attention-Deficit Disorder or Attention-Deficit/Hyperactivity Disorder in Children and Adolescents" (Bjorstad & Montgomery, 2005) and "Parent Training Interventions for Attention Deficit Hyperactivity Disorder (ADHD) in Children Aged 5 to 18 Years" (Zwi et al., 2011).

Not all clinical questions are so easily searched, so you may want to explore the Cochrane Library's advanced search option. This resource is also easily browsed, as it is divided into major topic areas, including schizophrenia, drugs and alcohol, tobacco addiction, depression, and anxiety. Stymied searchers can also use the contents of the CDSR, which include the citations of the RCTs examined and each review's expert search strategy, for tackling tough questions. For example, if your search does not locate a Cochrane Review that specifically answers your question but you did find a closely related review, take a look at the original research and the review's search strategy with an eye toward incorporating these citations and expert search terms into your own searches.

As mentioned previously, the Cochrane Library simultaneously searches EBP databases in addition to the CDSR. One of these related resources—the Cochrane Central Register of Controlled Trials (CENTRAL)—will be discussed in Chapter 4.

Campbell Collaboration Reviews of Interventions and Policy Evaluations

Established in 2000, the **Campbell Collaboration (C2)** is a non-profit group patterned on the Cochrane Collaboration. Like the Cochrane Collaboration, the C2 creates and maintains systematic reviews focused on but not limited to behavioral science evidence in the areas of education, social justice, and crime. These reviews, written by policymakers, educators, practitioners, and consumers, are contained in the C2 Library of Systematic Reviews. Reviewers are urged to update their reviews at least every 24 months.

Access to the C2 Library is free online at www.campbellcollaboration.org/lib/ and includes access to PDF versions of the full texts of systematic reviews. Once at this website, users can search the more than 120 reviews by title, author, and keywords. In this search, the Boolean operator OR automatically gets inserted between search terms if no other operator is specified.

 Skill Exercise 3-4

Consider a recent knowledge need that arose in your practice that you think would be answerable by a filtered information source. Formulate that knowledge need as a PICO question by identifying its key components: P, I, C, O. Using your PICO question, run your search in either the Cochrane Library or the C2 Library and sift through the resulting citations. How many citations did you retrieve? Did the search provide satisfactory information? If the resultant citations were off topic, what other search terms or databases might you try? If too many citations were retrieved, what limits might you apply?

Database of Abstracts of Reviews of Effects

The Database of Abstracts of Reviews of Effects (DARE), established in 1994 and produced by the UK National Health Service Centre for Reviews and Dissemination, is available free at www.crd. york.ac.uk/crdweb or with a subscription via the Cochrane Library. Unfortunately, as of 2015 it is no longer being updated. DARE entries will probably remain relevant through 2017, but will lose currency thereafter. Nonetheless, it contains over 13,000 structured abstracts that critically analyze systematic reviews culled from major biomedical databases, select journals, and a wide range of other literature. DARE reviews focus on investigating the impact of various healthcare and social care interventions, making it an effective resource for behavioral health and addiction questions; a few DARE abstracts also investigate diagnostic systematic reviews.

Each DARE review was written by two authors, who critically appraised each selected systematic review, providing a concise summary, including its funding sources, study design, results, and author conclusions. Reviewers also provided critical analysis of the strengths and weaknesses of each selected review; this was intended to help busy practitioners in making educated decisions about whether or not the particular systematic review is worth the time and effort to review in full. For practitioners interested in pursuing the original systematic review, DARE saves time by providing a direct link to the original review's citation in PubMed.

BMJ Clinical Evidence

BMJ Clinical Evidence is designed to aid practitioners in making evidence-based treatment decisions based on a summary of available evidence regarding the benefits and harms of a therapy. Available online and for mobile devices, this resource provides evidence for over 2,000 treatments and preventative measures for more than 200 common health conditions, including ones in behavioral health. The mental health section covers drug and alcohol misuse, depression in adults and children, post-traumatic stress disorder, and eating disorders, as well as other behavioral health topics. Available by subscription at www.clinicalevidence.com, this resource undergoes continual updating.

Clinicians or epidemiologists with significant EBP experience thoroughly analyze health conditions and their interventions for

BMJ Clinical Evidence. Each condition is presented as an easy-to-use comprehensive module. Each module contains the authors' systematic review of the health condition, which succinctly summarizes the benefits or disadvantages of the related interventions. These systematic reviews flow from current RCTs, observational studies, and other systematic reviews.

A major strength of *BMJ Clinical Evidence* lies in how it compiles all of this key information into one easy-to-access location. It also benefits from being a BMJ resource, meaning that it connects to the wide range of BMJ journals and evidence resources. This extensive connectivity allows users to quickly access additional information with minimal effort. Understand, though, that access to the full texts of these BMJ resources requires a user to have subscription access. One of the drawbacks of *BMJ Clinical Evidence* is that its focus on therapy makes it less useful for other types of clinical questions.

Each web page of *BMJ Clinical Evidence* features a standard search box, which is relatively user-friendly as long as you remember that OR is automatically inserted between all terms and that the Boolean operators AND and NOT must be capitalized. This resource does feature search help pages. In addition to searching via its search box, one can easily browse *BMJ Clinical Evidence* by section or health condition, arranged alphabetically.

Evidence-Based Journals

Journals dedicated to facilitating EBP have become a recent trend in publishing. Examples throughout healthcare include *Evidence-Based Complementary and Alternative Medicine*, *Evidence-Based Medicine*, the *International Journal of Evidence-Based Healthcare*, *Evidence-Based Nursing*, and the *Journal of Evidence-Based Dental Practice*. Most relevant for our purposes are journals in behavioral health and the addictions, such as *Evidence-Based Practice of Child and Adolescent Mental Health*, *Translational Behavioral Medicine*, *Journal of Evidence-Based Social Work*, and especially *Evidence-Based Mental Health*.

Evidence-Based Mental Health began in 1998 as a quarterly journal of structured abstracts that summarize and analyze behavioral health articles, including original studies and review articles from over 100 international medical journals and the Cochrane Library. Each structured abstract focuses on an individual article and succinctly presents its methods, main results, and conclusions. A mental health expert also provides a short critical analysis of the main article and makes recommendations for its use in clinical practice. A strength of *Evidence-Based Mental Health* is its value-added commentary, which can influence a practitioner's decision about whether or not to pursue the original article for further examination. This resource is useful because of its behavioral health focus and because it conveniently pulls together a wide range of key journal articles that would otherwise be difficult for a single practitioner to access and effectively analyze.

Evidence-Based Mental Health requires a subscription for access in print or online at ebmh.bmj.com. Electronic access provides the best option for browsing by issue or topic. Besides browsing *Evidence-Based Mental Health*, one can also run a keyword or title word search of the journal. To access these search options, click on "advanced search." This search assumes AND between your search terms, but you can also use OR or NOT to narrow a search. One can also input the citation of an original article to see if it has undergone appraisal in *Evidence-Based Mental Health*. This feature can be helpful if you are having difficulty tracking down the full text of a promising original article, since the *Evidence-Based Mental Health* abstract always provides a summary and a recommendation for practice.

In addition to EBP journals, many titles across a wide range of specialties now also include evidence sections, including meta-analyses of articles, systematic reviews, or evidence-based approaches to particular topics. For example, the *American Journal of Psychiatry* includes a monthly series called "Treatment in Psychiatry," which features a hypothetical clinical case that presents a common problem in patient care, summarizes the relevant literature, and includes expert recommendations for treatment and diagnosis. For another example, consult the journal *Psychiatric Services*; it often includes the column "Best Practices," which introduces a best practice based on research evidence and provides clinical commentary.

Key Terms

BMJ Clinical Evidence
Boolean operators
Campbell Collaboration (C2)
Cochrane Database of
  Systematic Reviews (CDSR)
eMedicine
filtered information sources

National Registry of Evidence-
  Based Programs and Practices
  (NREPP)
PICO
truncation
UpToDate
wild cards

Answers to Selected Skill Exercises

 Skill Exercise 3-1

Any of the following search strings would retrieve relevant articles:

> *depression AND non-response AND psychotherapy*
>
> *depression AND (non-response OR "maximum dosage" OR augment OR "treatment failure") AND psychotherapy*
>
> *depress* AND (non-response OR "maximum dosage" OR augment* OR "treatment failure") AND psychotherap**

* = truncation

Recommended Readings and Websites

Berke, D. M., Rozell, C. A., Hogan, T. P., Norcross, J. C., & Karpiak, C. P. (2011). What clinical psychologists know about evidence-based practice: Familiarity with online resources and research methods. *Journal of Clinical Psychology, 67*, 1–11.

Centre for Health Evidence, www.cche.net

Duke University Evidence-Based Practice, guides.mclibrary.duke.edu/ebm

EBM Resources for Mobile Devices, guides.library.upenn.edu/content.php?pid=192036&sid=1751087

How to Use the Cochrane Library, www.cochranelibrary.com/help/how-to-use-cochrane-library.html

Mesgari, M., Okoli, C., Mehdi, M., Nielsen, F. Å., & Lanamäki, A. (2015). "The sum of all human knowledge": A systematic review of scholarly research on the content of Wikipedia. *Journal of the Association for Information Science and Technology, 66*, 219–245.

Oxford University Cochrane Library Tutorial, learntech.physiol.ox.ac.uk/cochrane_tutorial/cochlibdoe4.php

University of Toronto Centre for Evidence-based Medicine, ktclearinghouse.ca/cebm/

4

Locating the Best Available Research: Unfiltered Sources

U NFILTERED INFORMATION SOURCES, LIKE PUBMED OR PsycINFO, offer the more traditional bibliographic sources. In the past, you were probably inclined to search these sites first. These sources contain "virtually everything" published, without filter or fetter. Unfiltered information exists in a wide variety of bibliographic databases and generally forms the basis for all other kinds of research evidence.

The huge weakness of unfiltered information is that it needs to be analyzed and synthesized, which will prove time-consuming. Can you realistically read the estimated 1,000 RCTs published each year in healthcare? Do you want to access and absorb each of PubMed's 341,861 articles on "depression" or PsycINFO's 54,882 entries on "autism" (as of February 2016)? Also, because so much unfiltered information exists, it can be quite difficult to search and isolate the key evidence related to a topic. That's why we and other experienced searchers begin with reliable filtered information (as summarized in Chapter 3) and turn to these unfiltered sources only when necessary.

Fortunately, filtered information sources all usually operate under the same search concepts, so a strong grasp of the search basics in Chapter 3 will make approaching any database less frustrating and time-consuming. In this chapter, however, we will introduce the concept of **controlled vocabularies** (e.g., Medical Subject Headings), which will prove particularly valuable when searching unfiltered resources.

Controlled Vocabularies

While searching the behavioral health and addiction literature, you will most likely encounter **Medical Subject Headings** (MeSH). These represent the National Library of Medicine's (NLM) subject heading system, or controlled vocabulary, which helps searchers generate comprehensive targeted searches in MEDLINE. Similar controlled vocabularies, offshoots of MeSH, have been adopted by other search systems such as CINAHL and PsycINFO. Bearing this in mind, a good grasp of MeSH fundamentals will help you to understand and use other controlled vocabularies.

One of the major benefits of searching with MeSH (or any controlled vocabulary) is that it provides a standardized way of describing a resource. A search with MeSH for "antidepressive agents," for example, will automatically retrieve information about the related terms "thymoleptics" and "antidepressant drugs," making it unnecessary to string synonyms together with OR. This approach is unlike keyword searching, in which using only the phrase "antidepressive agents" may miss relevant citations as a result of divergent vocabulary. Additionally, this keyword search may retrieve citations not specifically related to antidepressive agents. Remember: A keyword search generally scans only for the inputted string of letters, which does not guarantee that the citations retrieved will focus on your topic. Thus a keyword search for "antidepressive agents" might retrieve, for example, articles that simply state, "This article does not address antidepressive agents." Searching with MeSH helps avoid this problem thanks to the efforts of professional indexers, who scan each article and assign relevant MeSH terms based on the article's major concepts. Therefore when you search using MeSH, you will retrieve articles that specifically include the MeSH term, which helps to ensure extremely targeted retrieval.

Indexers are only human, and at times you may not agree with their indexing decisions. Thus if you have difficulty searching with MeSH, you may desire to try a keyword search to ensure that you do not miss any relevant citations. MeSH is updated annually. Between updates, however, new treatments and conditions emerge, and new medications get launched. Because these new concepts will not enter the system until the annual update, it is important to search for these concepts as keywords.

We now describe unfiltered information resources in more detail and present the frequent sources for each. These examples will illustrate but not exhaust sources in common use among behavioral health and addictions practitioners and researchers. As you will recall, unfiltered information comprises the "raw data" of original research studies that have not yet been synthesized or aggregated. Among the most popular unfiltered information sources for behavioral health and addictions practitioners are MEDLINE, PubMed Clinical Queries, CINAHL, Social Services Abstracts, PsycINFO, LexisNexis, the Cork Database, and Google Scholar.

MEDLINE

The premier database of the National Library of Medicine (NLM), **MEDLINE** currently contains over 22 million biomedical citations, dating back to 1946. MEDLINE indexes approximately 5,600 biomedical journals published in the United States and over 80 other countries. The strength of MEDLINE is its massive size and scope as well as its expert indexing with MeSH. Users can search MEDLINE free online or on mobile devices through **PubMed**, a larger database at www.pubmed.gov (described next).

Searching MEDLINE through PubMed also retrieves "PubMed only" citations not yet added to MEDLINE. Initially this broader retrieval may seem counterproductive, but because you want the most current information, MEDLINE in-process citations can be crucial. In-process MEDLINE citations generally consist of the most current research simply waiting to be incorporated into MEDLINE; the delay results in part from the time it takes to assign MeSH terms to each citation. Additionally, PubMed contains older citations that have not been incorporated into MEDLINE. These citations, although older, can sometimes prove critical (Perkins, 2001), so incorporating all of PubMed's citations into a search can yield better results.

At first glance, the PubMed search box appears standard. Behind the scenes, however, PubMed is shaping your search. For example, in Chapter 3, we described searching the Cochrane Database of Systematic Reviews to retrieve a couple of excellent Cochrane Reviews (filtered information on your clinical question of how family therapy compares with individual therapy for treating a child with ADHD, ODD, and family tension). Let's assume, however, that unfortunately, the filtered information you found simply did not answer your specific question. You decide to move to the final phase and search the larger, unfiltered literature.

 The companion website for this book presents color screenshots of the websites of all the unfiltered information sources (including PubMed) featured in this chapter.

A viable search could look like 'ADHD AND "family therapy."' This search query seems straightforward; however, PubMed actually creates a search that comprehensively combines MeSH and text words. For example, "ADHD" is searched as a keyword as well as by its proper MeSH, "attention deficit disorder with hyperactivity." "Family therapy," which is a MeSH, is also searched both as a MeSH and keyword. This search produced 1,015 results, which when searching for a quick EBP answer would overwhelm the reader. Using the "limits" available in the navigation bar on the left side of the screen, one can search specifically by age group, date, language, article types (including RCTs), and a host of other options. Remember to apply limits one at a time and to take care when selecting PubMed limits, because limits remain in effect until deselected. For example, if in the above search you had limited the age group to "child: 6–12" and subsequently decided to research your adult patient Francesco's condition, you would need to deselect the child age limit; otherwise, your search would retrieve only citations applicable to children.

Using one of the Cochrane Reviews that popped up earlier, a searcher could also identify several original studies within that review worth investigating further. For easy tracking of citations and full texts (when available) of these original articles, PubMed has a tool called the "Single Citation Matcher." This tool, located at the bottom of PubMed's home page, enables searchers to input full or partial citations in order to pull up the full record, which in some cases may include the article's abstract or even its full text. Note, however, that because Cochrane reviewers may select information outside of PubMed, the Single Citation Matcher does not always locate a citation for the original study in PubMed.

 Skill Exercise 4-1

Think of a recent patient, case, or consultation in which you found yourself wondering about the research evidence for a particular clinical decision. Formulate that into a knowledge need that you believe would be answerable by unfiltered information sources. Formulate that knowledge need as a PICO question by identifying its key components:

P -

I -

C -

O -

Question:

Using your PICO question, run your search strategy in PubMed and sift through the resulting citations. How overwhelming did you find the number of retrieved citations? What limits might you apply to return a smaller number of citations better directed at your exact knowledge need?

Now run the same search on one of the filtered information sources featured in Chapter 3 (for example, the Cochrane or the National Registry of Evidence-Based Programs and Practices). Take note of the huge difference in the number of citations (favoring the unfiltered source of PubMed) and probably the advantage in evidence-based guidance (favoring the filtered source of your choosing). That, in a nutshell, highlights the essential difference between unfiltered and filtered information sources: virtually everything published on a topic versus research summaries. Your choice!

PubMed Clinical Queries

PubMed Clinical Queries is a PubMed option geared specifically for practitioners seeking EBP answers. It appears on PubMed's home page or at www.ncbi.nlm.nih.gov/pubmed/clinical. PubMed Clinical Queries provides three search options: clinical study categories, systematic reviews, or medical genetics citations.

When searching PubMed Clinical Queries, the search box returns results from all three options, but you will most likely have interest in the Clinical Study Categories citations, featured on the far left. This option applies specialized search filters to your search. These filters can be seen in their entirety at www.ncbi.nlm.nih.gov/books/ NBK3827/#pubmedhelp.Clinical_Queries_Filters. Searches are basically conducted as they would be in PubMed, except that searchers are also prompted to select a search category, such as etiology, diagnosis, therapy, prognosis, or clinical prediction guides. Lastly, users select the scope of the returned citations by running either a "broad, sensitive search" or a "narrow, specific search." A broad, sensitive search returns more results (some of which may be off-topic), whereas a narrow, specific search locates fewer but more relevant citations. PubMed Clinical Queries offers a quick portal to clinically relevant citations but does not search the literature comprehensively.

One last note regarding PubMed: The NLM provides a great deal of high-quality online support for all of its resources, including interactive online tutorials, "frequently asked questions" pages, and help manuals. Also, one can find face-to-face PubMed trainings offered on occasion (see training schedules at nnlm.gov/ training-schedule).

 The companion website contains another practice example of searching both filtered and unfiltered databases to address a patient's question. See "The Case of Juliette."

Cumulative Index to Nursing and Allied Health Literature

The database **CINAHL** (Cumulative Index to Nursing and Allied Health Literature) contains over 4.8 million citations from 5,400 nursing and allied health journals, some dating back to 1937. This database's strength stems from its extensive coverage of nursing literature, as it includes the majority of English-language nursing journals and publications. Although some of its content overlaps with MEDLINE's, CINAHL is definitely the key resource for nursing literature. Also, it provides citations for books, chapters, conference proceedings, dissertations, newsletters, standards of practice, and research instruments, all of which would be extremely difficult to find elsewhere. Although primarily a bibliographic database, CINAHL does offer some full-text articles. Access requires an online subscription through the library vendor EBSCO (www.ebscohost.com/nursing/products/cinahl-databases/cinahl-complete). We performed the following search example using EBSCO's search platform.

After searching the filtered information and not finding a relevant resource, you have not answered the following clinical question about your patient Annique: For a 61-year-old with hot flashes, would treatment with soy improve her symptoms compared with no therapy? You decide to try CINAHL.

A viable search could look like ' "hot flashes" AND soy.' This simple keyword search looked for the specified terms in the title, subject heading, abstract, and instrumentation fields, returning 94 citations. This is a manageable number of citations to scan; however, you could also limit your search by applying a wide range of limits, including age group, publication type, date range, and language, that you will find in the left navigation bar. Another way to further target this search would involve searching by subject heading only; EBSCO's interface makes this easy, as it allows users to automatically map the search terms to the appropriate subject heading in the CINAHL thesaurus.

Social Services Abstracts

Geared toward professionals in social work, human services, and community development, Social Services Abstracts is available by subscription online through ProQuest at www.proquest.com. This database, produced by the National Association of Social Workers, provides access to bibliographic citations and abstracts from over 1,300 journals, dissertations, and book reviews dating back to 1965.

Citations are added monthly. Coverage highlights the following topics: social services and addictions, social and health policy, community and mental health services, family and social welfare, social work practice, and crisis intervention.

You can also search Social Services Abstracts using the ProQuest search interface, which presents you with a user-friendly search box. The search box accepts Boolean operators and allows for truncation. Directly under the search box you will find a link to additional search tips and an advanced search.

PsycINFO

A subscription database produced by the American Psychological Association (APA), **PsycINFO** provides access to mental and behavioral health information including journal articles, books, dissertations, and technical reports. PsycINFO contains over 4 million citations, many from 2,500 journals, 99% of which undergo peer review. It boasts an international scope and, in some cases, dates back to the 1890s. PsycINFO's major strength lies its behavioral health focus across a wide variety of indexed resources. PsycINFO primarily features citations and abstracts only; thus tracking down full-text resources takes valuable time. PsycINFO is available by subscription at www.PsycINFO.com or through vendors, including EBSCO. The following search examples come from the subscription EBSCO interface, which is used by many libraries, although other database vendors such as Ovid and ProQuest also provide access to PsycINFO.

The EBSCO search platform defaults to a basic search, which works fine for the majority of searches. This simple search interface allows use of the three major Boolean operators (AND, OR, NOT) and the application of key limits, such as publication type, age group, population group, and publication date. Apply limits with care and try to apply them one by one so that you can better track your search results.

After searching for filtered information regarding Annique's question about soy as a potential therapy for hot flashes, you still do not feel satisfied with your findings. You decide to try the unfiltered evidence. You start with PsycINFO.

A viable search could look like '"hot fl?shes" AND soy.' In addition to Boolean operators, this search uses a wild card, as indicated by "?." In this case, "?" would retrieve citations for both *hot flashes* and *hot flushes*. In PsycINFO, this search retrieved only 10 articles. Despite this small return, a search need not stop here, thanks to the database's "cited reference" feature, which links the user to information about articles cited by the articles retrieved. PsycINFO currently contains more than 23 million cited references, allowing you to connect to related citations and (in some cases) full text that may otherwise be difficult to find. The cited-reference feature often serendipitously leads to great evidence. Additionally, PsycINFO provides a "times cited in this database" link, which allows users to view any articles that have cited the original article.

To aid in your selection of search terms and to help you better target your search, PsycINFO uses the specialized *Thesaurus of Psychological Index Terms* (Tuleya, 2007); this consists of 8,400 standard and cross-referenced terms added to PsycINFO citations by APA's expert indexers. The EBSCO interface allows for both browsing and searching of the thesaurus. Once you have found an appropriate index term, you can manually insert it into the search box as a keyword. Users also have the option of specifically selecting index terms as descriptors for searches. When searched as a descriptor, the database will retrieve only citations that the APA indexers have specifically tagged with that particular term. This hand indexing allows for a more targeted search.

For example, "schizophrenia" searched as a keyword retrieves 113,032 citations. "Schizophrenia" searched as a descriptor retrieves 74,462 citations. Even when searched as the more targeted descriptor, this topic remains too large to be realistically searched. Therefore you may find it useful to take advantage of the option "Narrow results by subject: major heading" found in the resource's left navigation bar, to narrow the results to a subset of related topics. For the example of schizophrenia, "family therapy" and "neuroleptic drugs" are two of the narrowing options.

One might well expect that identical literature searches conducted on PsycINFO and PubMed would yield hugely overlapping results. One would be wrong. The two unfiltered search engines generate significantly different proportions of relevant articles overall and even with respect to particular mental disorders (Wu et al., 2012). The lesson is to search more than one unfiltered source, since their respective search strategies, decision points, syntaxes, subject headings, and databases probably differ.

Skill Exercise 4-2

Recently, a client mentioned her concern about the impact of bullying on her 8-year old son. Although her son did not directly experience bullying as a victim, she knows that he has witnessed bullying activities aimed at his classmates. Based on this scenario, formulate a PICO question. Identify the key components—P, I, C, O—and then formulate your question. List the search terms that you will use and how they would be combined using Boolean operators (AND/OR).

Run your search strategy in PsycINFO and sift through the resulting citations. How many citations did you retrieve? Too many, right? If the resultant citations drifted off topic, what other search terms or databases might you try? Since you retrieved too many citations, what limits might you apply? This exercise should assist you in delimiting your future searches on unfiltered sources and will probably demonstrate the simultaneous benefits and disadvantages of searching the world's largest psychology bibliographic database.

LexisNexis

Available by subscription at www.lexisnexis.com, LexisNexis provides access to over 5,800 full-text publications. These publications include more than a thousand world newspapers, magazines, and broadcast transcripts along with a wide variety of legal information sources, including court decisions, federal regulations, and international legislation. LexisNexis is an extremely powerful search tool that offers special utility because it aggregates and makes searchable materials that would otherwise prove extremely difficult to locate and search.

This benefit of LexisNexis is especially true of the case of locating information from the media. For example, if in passing a colleague mentions that she had recently viewed a short television news segment on soy as a treatment for hot flashes, finding the specific segment would constitute an arduous task without LexisNexis, which maintains full-text records of transcripts of sources of this type. Additionally, LexisNexis is invaluable for locating legal information, because it brings together in a single resource many disparate legal resources, such as codes and regulations, case law, and information from law reviews and legal magazines.

LexisNexis features a simple interface that searches across news, legal, and business publications. For example, suppose you practice in Massachusetts and are interested in recent legal cases dealing with the civil commitment of patients. An appropriate search string could begin with "civil commitment!" Notice that one need not include the Boolean operator AND, because it is automatically inserted between all search terms, and that the wild card "!" was added to capture the plural form of commitment. OR will also work in this database, but you must include it between the appropriate terms.

The search for "civil commitment!" returns 987 results. However, because your interest focuses on legal information for Massachusetts, you would select the geography link from the left navigation bar. The link enables you to limit your search to a region or state. Limiting the search to Massachusetts returns 23 relevant citations.

Cochrane Central Register of Controlled Trials

The Cochrane Central Register of Controlled Trials (CENTRAL), accessed via the Cochrane Library (www.cochranelibrary.com), currently contains over 489,000 citations for controlled clinical trials and studies of healthcare interventions gathered by search professionals from biomedical databases (primarily MEDLINE and Embase), specialized registers, and conference proceedings. Citations include each study's title, location, date of publication, and in some cases a short summary, but not the full text. The primary use of this database is compiling systematic reviews for the filtered Cochrane Database of Systematic Reviews (CDSR), but it can also be useful for finding citations of studies that you could investigate further to answer your question. You would search CENTRAL using the same approach as for the CDSR, described in Chapter 3.

Cork Database

Begun as a medical education initiative at the Dartmouth School of Medicine, the Cork Database provides access to over 120,000 citations on substance abuse taken from professional journals, books, and reports from federal and state agencies. It is available free at www. projectcork.org. Unfortunately, as of 2014, this database is no longer being updated; however, its existing contents provide access to information from the social sciences and life sciences as well as from clinical settings, with special attention paid to coverage of substance abuse, college and university campuses, treatment methods, and the impact of substance abuse on society. The Cork database should remain relevant for a few more years but will thereafter become obsolete.

Google Scholar

Accessible free of cost at www.scholar.google.com, **Google Scholar** searches "scholarly sources" including journal articles, book chapters, graduate theses, institutional repositories, and conference proceedings across many disciplines, including the health sciences. Google Scholar provides access to citations and, for some unrestricted publications, full texts. Of course, you may gain additional access to full texts through your affiliated library. Note that performing an ordinary Google search does not do a Google Scholar search; you must specifically go to Google Scholar.

Two of the most attractive features of Google Scholar are its ease of use and its ability to provide lots of citations (perhaps too many citations) almost immediately. However, Google Scholar does not specify which resources it includes, nor does it define what criteria it uses when labeling a resource "scholarly." These limitations could mean that information not generally considered scholarly may be included in search results or that scholarly sources may be excluded.

Let's work a search example about a potential relationship between Francesco's lack of medical insurance and his recurring depression. Out of curiosity, you run a Google Scholar Search. A viable search could read, "Does not having medical insurance contribute to depression?"

Unlike the other information resources discussed thus far, the basic search feature of Google Scholar allows the use of natural language. By default, Google Scholar automatically inserts the Boolean operator AND between all search terms. To use OR, you must type OR in capital letters.

Although the basic Google Scholar interface is useful, it may be more beneficial to search using the advanced search feature accessed by clicking on the small inverted triangle near the right edge of the

---

Box 4.1 Featured Unfiltered Information Resources

- PubMed (MEDLINE): www.pubmed.gov
- PubMed Clinical Queries: www.ncbi.nlm.nih.gov/pubmed/clinical
- Cumulative Index to Nursing and Allied Health Literature (CINAHL): www.cinahl.com or at www.ebsco.com
- PsycINFO: www.PsycINFO.com or www.ebsco.com
- LexisNexis: www.lexisnexis.com
- Cochrane Central Register of Controlled Trials (CENTRAL): www.cochranelibrary.com
- Social Services Abstracts: www.proquest.com
- Cork Database: www.projectcork.org
- Google Scholar: www.scholar.google.com

---

search box. In the advanced search mode, you can search for exact phrases, exclude words, and limit the search by date, author, or publication title. Users can also select to restrict searches to just the titles of articles, thereby returning a very targeted set of results.

For a list of featured unfiltered information resources, please see Box 4.1.

 Skill Exercise 4-3

Consider again your PICO question about bullying from the previous skill exercise (4-2). Conduct the same search in Google Scholar as you did in PsycINFO. Compare the search results from the two unfiltered sources. What similarities and differences do you detect between the retrieved citations?

Evidence-Based Practice Search Engines

A final type of information resource does not fall gracefully into any of the categories of background, filtered, or unfiltered information. Evidence-based practice search engines simultaneously enable access to all three types of resources. The free **TRIP** (Turning Research Into Practice) database (www.tripdatabase.com) is an excellent example of an EBP search engine, because it quickly retrieves practice guidelines, websites, systematic reviews, evidence synopses, and journal citations in a single search. It seeks to become the one-stop shopping site for EBP research resources.

Updated frequently, the TRIP database contains evidence-based synopses like *BMJ Clinical Evidence*, clinical guidelines, systematic reviews, core medical journals such as the *New England Journal of Medicine*, and links to "canned" searches in PubMed, which allow users to run PubMed Clinical Queries designed for their research topics. Keep in mind, however, that even though the TRIP database may list citations from certain subscription resources, you must still have subscription access to obtain the full texts of these restricted resources.

The TRIP database is a commercial site featuring advertising, which raises the possibility of external influence by its advertisers, which prominently include the pharmaceutical industry. Users can purchase a TRIP premium account, which removes advertising and makes available certain TRIP features, such as its advanced search.

The TRIP database is easy to use. However, you will need to think more carefully about your search terms than you do for general Web searching, once again isolating the key concepts you wish to search. Imagine that you are approaching the following question for the first time: "For an 8-year-old with ADHD, ODD, and family tension, would family therapy or individual therapy be the treatment of choice?" A viable search for this search engine would be as follows: 'ADHD AND "family therapy."' Notice that we use quotation marks to alert the system to search "family therapy" as a phrase.

In TRIP, it is unnecessary to include multiple synonyms to ensure comprehensiveness, because the database automatically uses a synonym dictionary to include related terms. In the search described above, for example, "ADHD" also includes "attention-deficit/hyperactivity disorder" and several other synonyms. You can also view the synonyms used from the results page.

The TRIP database displays for each citation the title, the source of the information, the publication date, and, when available, its level of evidence. In the right-hand navigation bar the results are broken up into several key filter areas, such as evidence-based synopses, guidelines (broken out by region), systematic reviews, e-textbooks, patient decision aids, and clinical questions. The MEDLINE results are also broken out by the main question types (e.g., diagnosis, therapy, or prognosis). Clicking on the PubMed Clinical Queries links dumps you into the PubMed search interface for that search.

Because TRIP connects users with various types of information sources that all use different search systems, you sacrifice precision and control over the search when using it. In some cases, this will mean getting inundated by too many resources. Although this resource aims to be extremely comprehensive, several gaps persist. You may not find coverage of some specialty journals that would appear using other, more specialized resources.

Accessing Information on Tests and Measures

Last but not least, we turn to the more specialized matter of locating evidence on behavioral tests and measures. Virtually all research studies in behavioral health use tests or measures. Most importantly, tests often define the dependent variable(s) in a study. For example, tests may operationalize levels of depression, ADHD, alcoholism, or hot flashes. Test results may also describe characteristics of the participants in a study, for example, their levels of academic achievement. Because of the central role played by tests and measures, thoughtful evaluation of research requires accessing information about them.

Some research reports provide detailed information about the tests employed in the study—for example, regarding their development, reliability, and validity. However, such information often does not appear. Research reports typically provide little information beyond the name of the test and reference to its manual. In fact, sometimes you may find a test referred to only by its acronym or initials. Even when researchers provide test information on such matters as reliability and validity, you need to think critically about the test. The researchers are not an unbiased source of information. Having selected a test, they are certainly inclined to say that it is a reliable and valid measure rather than providing a long list of its limitations (which all tests have). In many cases, then, you need to secure additional information about the test or measure.

We identify here the most immediately helpful sources and then provide references to additional sources.

Test Information Databases

The Educational Testing Service **(ETS) Test Collection**, Web-accessible at www.ets.org/test_link/about, provides descriptive information for approximately 25,000 tests. (If the Web address given here does not work, just enter "ETS Test Collection" in any Internet search engine.) Once at the site, click on "Find a Test" on the left side of the screen, then "Search the Test Link database" in the middle of the screen. The ETS Test Collection is searchable by test title, author, keywords (e.g., anxiety), and even acronym (e.g., BDI will locate the Beck Depression Inventory as well as several other tests with the initials BDI in their titles, and STAI will locate the State Trait Anxiety Inventory).

For most purposes, the default "Basic Search" tab works well. The "Advanced Search" tab allows for more targeted searching. The initial search (e.g., using BDI) returns bare-bones information: test title, author, and publication year. Clicking on the test title link brings up more information, including a brief abstract about the test's purpose, target group, and publisher or other source (e.g., a journal article where the test first appeared). Knowing the publisher becomes crucial for using another source of information, the publisher's catalog, as described later in this chapter.

The major strengths of the ETS Test Collection lie in its immediate accessibility on the Internet and its comprehensiveness: It attempts to capture every behavioral test available in English. The principal drawback is that it does not provide evaluative information about the test. The best and the worst get equal coverage and are indistinguishable in terms of quality. Another drawback concerns its currency: It does not always have information about the latest versions of tests.

A source somewhat similar to the ETS Test Collection is the Health and Psychosocial Instruments (HaPI) database, a product of Behavioral Measurement Database Services. You will find it available as an EBSCOhost database. The product must be purchased separately and is not free on the Internet.

A hard-copy counterpart to the ETS Test Collection is *Tests in Print* (TIP; Anderson et al., 2016). Now in its ninth edition, with new editions appearing about every three years, TIP attempts to list all tests regularly published and in English; it has approximately 3,000 entries. Like the ETS Test Collection, this hard-copy source provides only basic information about tests: purpose, scores, publisher, target audience, administrative format, and so on. It does not provide evaluations of quality. It is quite comprehensive for regularly published tests but does not include unpublished tests. For regularly published tests it tends to be more up to date than the ETS Test Collection. Its major drawback is simply that it is hard copy and hence must be found in a library (most academic libraries will have a copy) and be searched by hand.

Launched in 2011 by the APA, the **PsycTESTS** database concentrates on tests not available from commercial publishers. Entries come directly from authors, journal articles, dissertations, and similar sources. Over 30,000 entries are now posted, with many of the instruments immediately available for use via download from PsycTESTS. However, the database's utility remains unclear, as it is still in development. Like PsycINFO and PsycABSTRACTS, PsycTESTS requires a subscription (for additional information, see www.apa.org/pubs/databases/psyctests/index.aspx).

Test Reviews

None of the aforementioned sources provides evaluative information about tests. The premier source devoted to providing such professional evaluation is the *Mental Measurements Yearbook* (Carlson et al., 2017), now in its 20th edition, with new editions appearing about every three years. This source is often referred to by its initials, **MMY**, or as **Buros**, after its originator, Oscar Buros. Experts in the field review evidence about a test's quality, defined primarily in terms of validity, reliability, norms, and practicality. MMY limits entries to regularly published tests. It has helpful indexes permitting searches by test title, test author, constructs, and names of scores. Each volume of MMY covers approximately 400 tests and provides two independent reviews for most entries. For a sample review in MMY, go to buros.org/review-samples.

All volumes of MMY appear in hard copy; major academic libraries have these volumes. The earliest volumes were available only in hard copy. Reviews appearing in the 10th edition of MMY (1989) and onward exist electronically in two forms. First, you can purchase a review via the Internet from the Buros Center for Testing (www.buros.org). This is much like shopping at the Amazon or L.L.Bean websites. The current cost runs $15 per review. Second, many academic libraries subscribe to an EBSCO host service that provides full MMY reviews at no cost to the user. An odd feature of searching within that database is that even when an exact test title is entered as the search term, the database sometimes returns not only that test but a host of related tests.

The major strength of MMY lies in its provision of professional reviews of test quality. Its major weakness is that it does not cover all tests. In addition, one must remember that the reviews are only opinions and are usually directed at the ordinary use of a test, whereas in a particular research study the test might be deployed in a different way. Finally, the reviewing process understandably takes some time to complete; thus, reviews are not always as up to date as one might hope.

Test Publishers

Most, but not all, of the tests used in research are available from a publisher, which can become a valuable source of information. The test information published in catalogs issued periodically in hard copy and on publishers' websites undergoes continual updates. These sites are easily located with any common search engine. Once located, these sites usually allow for easy searching to get to the test of interest.

Publishers' websites (or hard-copy catalogs) are the preferred sources of information about practical matters related to tests, such as current costs, new editions, recent technical manuals, types of response formats available, and so on. The other sources discussed above often have outdated information on these matters. However, do *not* consider the publisher a preferred source of information about the quality of a test, since the publisher has a vested interest in marketing and selling the test.

An Example

While working with Annique and her chronic depression, you come across in the unfiltered information an abstract of an article that provides relevant treatment research. The abstract contains reference to the RHRSD as the crucial outcome measure in the study. The initials do not ring a bell. You go to the Buros website (www.buros. org), click on the tab "Test Reviews and Information," then "Test Reviews Online," enter "RHRSD" under keywords for acronym search, and then click "Search." You learn that RHRSD stands for the Revised Hamilton Rating Scale for Depression and that the MMY contains two reviews of the RHRSD, which you can purchase online or access free through a university library. You also check the ETS Test Collection (www.ets.org/test_link/about), searching on the name of the test, and find that there are actually two versions of the RHRSD: the Clinician Rating Form, and the Self-Report Problem Inventory. Both the Buros site and the ETS Test Collection give Western Psychological Services as the RHRSD publisher. You search the Internet for Western Psychological Services, bring up its website (www.wpspublish.com), use the search function to locate the test, and get the publisher's information about scores, scoring services, and the like. Altogether, you have invested about 15 minutes getting a pretty good idea of what the RHRSD is all about.

 Skill Exercise 4-4

Access the ETS Test Collection at www.ets.org/test_link/about. On the right, click on "Search Test Link Database." In the Search box, enter a keyword, for example, depression, suicidal ideation, or any other keyword(s) you wish. Then, push Return or Enter.

You will get a list of tests relevant for your keyword(s). Test titles appear in blue. Put your cursor on one of the titles and left-click. Now you will get basic information about this test and information about its source (e.g., publisher), which you can follow up for more information.

Now try another search term or two. You can use another keyword, a test title, or a test acronym.

More Expert Assistance

This and the previous chapter have introduced you to popular unfiltered and filtered information resources for behavioral health, addictions, and healthcare and provided you with the fundamental skills to approach these resources as a searcher. Even with these skills and the increasing ease of scholarly searches, at times you will probably come up against a clinical question that proves difficult to answer. This situation may require specialized searching methods or niche resources. When this happens, your best bet is to contact a librarian at your local university or at your regional healthcare library.

Key Terms

Buros
CINAHL
controlled vocabularies
ETS Test Collection
Google Scholar
Medical Subject Headings
MEDLINE

*Mental Measurements
  Yearbook* (MMY)
PsycINFO
PsycTESTS
PubMed
TRIP
unfiltered information sources

Recommended Readings and Websites

Calhoun, C. D. (2013, October). Finding what you need: Tips for using PsycINFO effectively. *Psychological Science Agenda*. www.apa.org/science/about/psa/2013/10/using-psycinfo.aspx

Centre for Evidence-Based Mental Health, www.cebmh.com

ETS Test Collection, www.ets.org/test_link

Evidence-Based Behavioral Practice, www.ebbp.org

Hogan, T. P. (2013). Sources of information about psychological tests. In G. P. Koocher, J. C. Norcross, & B. A. Greene (Eds.), *Psychologist's desk reference* (3rd ed., pp. 145–147). New York, NY: Oxford University Press.

Maggio, L. A., Tannery, N. H., & Kanter, S. L. (2011). AM last page: How to perform an effective database search. *Academic Medicine, 86*(8), 1057.

PubMed Tutorial, www.nlm.nih.gov/bsd/disted/pubmedtutorial/cover.html

Searching for Evidence, www.ebbp.org/course_outlines/searching_for_evidence/

Shariff, S. Z., Bejaimal, S. A., Sontrop, J. M., Iansavichus, A. V., Haynes, R. B., Weir, M. A., & Garg, A. X. (2013). Retrieving clinical evidence: A comparison of PubMed and Google Scholar for quick clinical searches. *Journal of Medical Internet Research, 15*(8), e164.

5

Reading and Interpreting
the Research: Research Designs

E VIDENCE-BASED PRACTICE DEPENDS ON RESEARCH AS its key source of evidence. The research follows one of several designs, each with its own strengths and weaknesses. Each research study typically pursues one or more hypotheses. To understand and apply the research, we must focus on the way in which hypotheses are stated and on the characteristics of the research design. This chapter treats these topics.

Hypotheses: Research and Statistical

Most empirical studies include explicit hypotheses. These can prove a source of great confusion, because the typical study includes two distinct, even opposite, hypotheses. First comes the **research hypothesis**, also sometimes called the *scientific hypothesis*. The research hypothesis states what the researcher hopes or expects to show. In clinical contexts, a research hypothesis might read that "this new psychotherapy will benefit clients, specifically by reducing their depression."

Second comes the **statistical hypothesis**. The statistical hypothesis will virtually always state some version of the **null hypothesis** (described next). In our clinical example, the null hypothesis asserts that the new therapy does *not* work. In effect, the researcher hopes to reject the null hypothesis, thus confirming the research hypothesis (at a certain level of probability). A statistically significant result constitutes rejection of the null hypothesis. A nonsignificant result means we must retain the null hypothesis, thus disconfirming the research hypothesis. Because the phrasing of the research hypothesis and the statistical hypothesis typically "go in opposite directions," you must remain especially alert when reading research reports as to what hypothesis the authors mean when they make statements such as "the hypothesis was confirmed" or "the hypothesis was rejected."

 Skill Exercise 5-1

We have devised a new behavioral technique for dealing with hyperactivity in children. We plan to conduct a study to show its effectiveness in comparison with no treatment. Label the new behavioral treatment B and no treatment N. Use symbols to state the null hypothesis.

Null Hypothesis Significance Tests

After descriptive statistics (especially the mean, standard deviation, and correlation coefficient), the **null hypothesis significance test (NHST)** is the most common statistical technique encountered in the research literature. Despite numerous calls for curtailment or elimination of the NHST, it remains a prominent feature of behavioral health research. Many specific NHSTs exist (e.g., t, F, and χ^2), but they all share a few key properties, which we outline here.

First, as suggested by their name, all NHSTs start with some version of the null hypothesis.

Second, the hypothesis focuses on parameters of the population. We do not make hypotheses about statistics based on samples. We just calculate the statistics. In the language of inferential statistics, we customarily designate parameters with Greek letters. These parameters include μ (mu, or the mean), σ (sigma, or the standard deviation), and ρ (rho, or the correlation coefficient). Note that in most typefaces the Greek letter ρ looks like the English lowercase "p." But Greek ρ is not a "*p*," and you should not confuse it with the ubiquitous "*p*" used for probability statements in inferential statistics. When referencing more than one population, subscripts distinguish the respective parameters; for example, μ_1 and μ_2 refer to the means of population 1 and population 2, respectively. Alternatively, you may find subscripts that use English letters as initials for words describing the populations; for example, μ_T and μ_C might designate population means for treatment and control groups, respectively.

A third feature of NHSTs is that treatment research typically pits one condition against another (e.g., a psychotherapy condition vs. a control or no-treatment condition) or several conditions against one another (e.g., psychodynamic therapy vs. medication vs. control). A typical expression of a null hypothesis in these contexts is $\mu_1 = \mu_2$; that is, if we tested everyone in populations 1 and 2, we would find the population means to be equal. By a simple rearrangement of terms, $\mu_1 = \mu_2$ becomes $\mu_1 - \mu_2 = 0$, a pure expression of the null (zero) hypothesis. Some other examples of null hypotheses include the following:

- The correlation between anxiety and depression is the same (no difference) in males and females: $\rho_M = \rho_F$ (or $\rho_M - \rho_F = 0$).
- The variance in attention span is the same (no difference) in boys and girls: $\sigma_B^2 = \sigma_G^2$ (or $\sigma_B^2 - \sigma_G^2 = 0$).
- Using a solution-focused therapy, there is no difference in outcome whether there are one, two, three, or four therapy sessions: $\mu_1 = \mu_2 = \mu_3 = \mu_4$.

A fourth feature of NHSTs involves examination of statistics. The relevant statistics correspond to the parameters in the hypothesis. Thus, if the hypothesis involves population means, the relevant statistics are sample means. If the hypothesis involves a population correlation coefficient, the relevant statistic is a sample correlation coefficient.

Fifth, the statistics have a certain degree of instability, because they originate with samples drawn from the population, and every sample will likely differ somewhat from every other sample. We call this instability *sampling fluctuation* or *sampling variability*.

Sixth, a key part of any NHST entails the **standard error of a statistic**. The standard error of a statistic is the standard deviation of a distribution of sample statistics around its parent population parameter. We refer to the distribution of these statistics as the *sampling distribution*. (See Figure 6.3 for an illustration of a sampling distribution.)

Seventh, we have convenient, well-known formulas for most of the standard errors of statistics we use in hypothesis testing. An important feature of the standard errors of statistics is that sample size(s), usually notated as n or n_1, n_2, . . . , always enters into the denominator of the standard error. Thus as sample size (n) increases, the standard error decreases, and in small samples, the standard error increases.

Finally, NHST involves setting an **alpha level** (α), also known as a **significance level**. The most common levels are .05 and .01. Selection of any particular alpha level arises purely from historical convention. A researcher may use any alpha level. Whatever alpha level we adopt, if the result of the NHST is less than the designated alpha level, we declare the result statistically significant and reject the null hypothesis. Alternatively, we may express the result as an exact p value, which expresses the probability of obtaining the result by chance (as a result of random sampling variability) under the assumption that the null hypothesis holds true. This matter of alpha levels reminds us that NHST methodology always results in statements of probability, not certainty. We can say that a hypothesis proved "probably true" or "probably not true." We cannot say the hypothesis is "true" or "false."

Objections to Null Hypothesis Significance Testing

Statistical experts have voiced numerous (and often passionate) objections to NHST (Kline, 2011; Waserstein & Lazar, 2016; Wilkinson & APA Task Force on Statistical Inference, 1999). We note here only the two most prominent objections.

First, every null hypothesis will almost certainly prove false. Consider the hypothesis from above: $\rho_M = \rho_F$ (i.e., the correlation between anxiety and depression is the same in males and females). If ρ_M is .46 and ρ_F is .47, the null hypothesis proves false, albeit trivially so. We could make a similar case for any null hypothesis.

Second, the result of a NHST (reject or do not reject, significant or nonsignificant) depends excessively on sample size(s). With large samples, you can rather easily get "significant" or "highly significant" results. In contrast, small sample sizes will usually yield results of "no significant difference."

Two recommendations usually accompany the objections to NHST. The first suggests using **confidence intervals** (for statistics) either in place of or as an adjunct to NHST. The second suggests reporting measures of **effect size**. We cover both of these topics in the next chapter. The *Publication Manual of the American Psychological Association* (APA, 2010b) strongly urges that confidence intervals and measures of effect size accompany any tests of statistical significance.

Types of Error in Hypothesis Testing

Research studies make frequent reference to types of error (Type I and Type II) and to power in hypothesis testing in the context of NHST. Figure 5.1 defines types of errors in hypothesis testing. Constructing this figure requires us to play a mind game, pretending that we "know the true state of nature." In research we never know the true state of nature; if we did, we would not have to conduct the research. In the top row of Figure 5.1, we assume that we really do know the true state of nature, specifically, that we know the truth or falsity of the null hypothesis.

Let us use this scenario to develop the figure. We wish to determine if behavioral training in impulse control will prove useful for treating ADHD cases in elementary school children, like Jonathon. We have a pool of 100 boys identified as having ADHD in one school system. We randomly assign 50 boys to the behavioral training (B) group and assign the other 50 to the control condition (C). We measure improvement with the ADHD Combined index of the Conners 3 Teacher rating scale (Conners 3-T).

We begin with the usual null hypothesis: $\mu_B = \mu_C$, or $\mu_B - \mu_C = 0$, where the subscripts B and C stand for behavioral training and control, respectively. Examine each quadrant in Figure 5.1. The upper right quadrant represents the situation where the null hypothesis proved false (behavioral training really does work effectively), and our statistical test led to rejecting the null hypothesis, a correct conclusion. The upper left quadrant represents the situation where the null hypothesis proved true (behavioral training does not work) but

True State of Nature
for $\mu_B = \mu_C$

		It's True*	It's False**
Reject		Type I Error (prob = alpha)	Correct
Retain		Correct	Type II Error (prob = beta)

Conclusion based on statistical test { Reject / Retain

* μ_B really is equal to μ_C, that is, behavioral training is not effective.

** μ_B really is not equal to μ_C, that is, behavioral training is effective.

FIGURE 5.1 Types of errors in hypothesis testing.

our statistical test rejected the null hypothesis, yielding a "significant" result and indicating that behavioral training is effective—a finding that no doubt would be followed in the corresponding report by recommendations for adoption of this method. But the conclusion is in error, specifically a **Type I error**. One of the nice things about the NHST apparatus involves knowing the probability of making a Type I error. It is precisely alpha. We know, for example, that if we set $\alpha = .05$, there is a 5% chance that we will incorrectly reject the null hypothesis, even if it is exactly true.

We can, of course, reduce the chance of making a Type I error by setting alpha at a lower value, moving it, say, from .05 to .01. As we will show later, there is a drawback to this strategy. Probably the more important antidote to making a Type I error involves replicating the study several times in different settings before issuing treatment recommendations based on the results.

The Type I error rate applies to a single hypothesis test in a study. If we are testing hypotheses on more than one variable (as commonly happens in research studies), the chances of making a Type I error on at least one of the hypothesis tests increase. For example, if we conduct two tests with alpha set at .05, the probability of making a Type I error on the first test equals .05. The probability of making a Type I error on either the first test or the second test or on both tests runs higher than .05. This compounding of probabilities gets progressively worse as we conduct more hypothesis tests; it becomes particularly severe when we conduct a great many separate tests. For example, if we conduct 15 separate hypothesis tests with alpha at .05, the chance of making a Type I error somewhere among the entire set of tests is 50:50.

The **Bonferroni correction** adjusts the alpha value so that it accurately reflects the probability of making a Type I error. This correction involves dividing the original alpha level by the number of tests to be conducted and using the result as the adjusted or corrected alpha level. For example, if you want to work at an alpha of .05 but you are conducting 10 independent hypothesis tests, set alpha at .05/10 = .005; if you are conducting 20 statistical hypothesis tests, set alpha at .05/20 = .0025.

The book's companion website contains a worksheet giving Bonferroni corrections for α = .05 and .01 for 1–20 hypothesis tests. The formulas built into the worksheet enable you to substitute other alpha values and different numbers of statistical tests.

Skill Exercise 5-2

Continuing with our example of comparing a new behavioral treatment (B) with a control condition (C), suppose you have four measures of outcome. You want to operate at the .05 level of significance. Use the Bonferroni correction worksheet on the book's website to determine what alpha level you should use for your four tests so that you really operate at the .05 level.

Now consider the lower left quadrant in Figure 5.1. This represents the situation in which the null hypothesis is true (behavioral training is not effective), and the statistical test results in retaining (some prefer to say "not rejecting") the null hypothesis. This is a correct decision.

Finally, consider the lower right quadrant. The null hypothesis is false: Behavioral training really does work effectively. However, our statistical test failed to reject the null hypothesis; that is, we failed to detect a real difference. We might now abandon behavioral training and tell others that we tried it and it did not work. This is a **Type II error**: failing to reject the null hypothesis when we should reject it.

The probability of making a Type I error equals alpha. We designate the probability of making a Type II error as beta (β). We define the **power** of the statistical test as $1 - \beta$. This is the probability of *avoiding* a Type II error. The conventional goal for power is .80 (i.e., we have an 80% chance of correctly rejecting a false null hypothesis). In our example, $\beta = .80$ would mean we have an 80% chance of correctly identifying behavioral training as having a positive effect.

The Type II error constitutes one of the most pernicious in research studies. It may occur for many different reasons. We noted above that we can adjust the probability of making a Type I error by changing alpha. We can also adjust the probability of making a Type II error, but that adjustment involves many factors, which we now consider.

Power and Factors Affecting It

The greater the power of a statistical test, the less the probability of making a Type II error. Numerous ways exist to increase the power of a statistical test.

We continue with the example of contrasting behavioral training with a control condition for ADHD using 50 patients in each group. The null hypothesis states that no difference exists between the behavioral training and control groups. What factors in the structure of the statistical test (e.g., a *t*-test) will lead to rejecting the null hypothesis? Here are six ways to increase the power of a statistical test.

1. Increasing sample size magnifies the test statistic (e.g., *t* or *F*) by decreasing the standard error in the test. The size of samples is the most common concern in discussions of statistical power. A host of algorithms available on the Internet can determine the number of cases needed in each group to achieve a certain degree of power for a given effect size and alpha level or determine the power with a given number of cases, alpha level, and effect size.

 The book's companion website contains hyperlinks to several Internet sites that provide calculations for power and sample size.

2. Increasing the difference between the two conditions, for example, between behavioral training and control, magnifies t or F. You might wonder how to influence the difference between the means of two groups. In our study of the effectiveness of behavioral training, we have to ensure that the treatment has sufficient potency. We might call this the "wallop" or dosing factor. A treatment may prove effective if applied regularly over a 6-month period but ineffective if applied over a 6-day period.

3. Increasing the alpha level increases the likelihood that the statistical test will prove significant, yielding a more powerful test. For example, changing the alpha level from .01 to .05 makes it easier to find significance. Of course, this also increases the chance of making a Type I error. Setting the alpha level always involves a trade-off between Type I and Type II errors.

4. A related factor concerns use of a one-tailed rather than a two-tailed test. A one-tailed test provides greater power (provided the result occurs in the predicted direction). However, theoretical reasons suggest eschewing a one-tailed test. For example, to use a one-tailed test in a treatment study, one needs to make the gratuitous (and empirically unsupportable) assumption that the treatment could only prove beneficial and has no chance of causing harm.

5. Reducing the size of the standard deviations increases the likelihood that the statistical test will prove significant, making for a more powerful test. We can reduce the standard deviation size by using more homogeneous groups, for example, by restricting the age levels in the study and controlling other such variables. Of course, such restriction reduces the generalizability of the results, but it does increase power.

6. Using more reliable tests for the dependent variable increases the power of the statistical test. In our example, we use a test of ADHD. The impact of the reliability of the dependent measure on power is substantial (Baugh, 2001). In this regard, one must pay particular attention to tests of significance on subscales, which often have substantially less reliability than the full scales within which they reside. Researchers often overlook the effect of reliability when discussing power and effect size.

Several additional factors affect the power of a study's design, but the foregoing six illustrate the importance of the concept. All of these matters related to power prove very important for the researcher planning a study. However, they also hold importance for the person evaluating and applying research. Lack of appropriate power in research evaluating treatments may mean that a potentially effective treatment goes undetected. Conversely, in a large, multisite study with hundreds of patients, a statistically significant but small difference may not be of clinical import at all.

 Skill Exercise 5-3

Suppose you intend to conduct a study (an RCT) comparing the effectiveness of two treatments for social anxiety. On your outcome measure (a self-report test of anxiety, where a high score indicates high anxiety), you expect about a 5-point difference in mean scores between the two groups, say 50 versus 45, with a standard deviation of 10. You expect to have 20 cases in each group. What is the power of your statistical hypothesis test (where you set the statistical hypothesis as the usual null hypothesis, i.e., no difference)?

Access this website: stat.ubc.ca/~rollin/stats/ssize/ index.html. Click on the link for "Comparing Means for Two Independent Samples" and then click the button for "Calculate Power (for specified Sample Size)." Enter these values: For mu1, 50; for mu2, 45; for sigma (standard deviation), 10, for sample size, 20. Then click on "Calculate."

The result: Your power is only .35. You are not likely to reject the null hypothesis even if it is false. Either increase your sample size or don't waste your time doing the study. You can use the site to determine how large a sample you would need to reach the "industry standard" of .80 for power. Click on the button for "Calculate Sample Size."

Try out some other values on the website.

Test Statistics Commonly Used in Null Hypothesis Significance Testing

Null hypothesis significance tests commonly use three types of test statistics: t, F, and χ^2. When the NHST involves comparing one sample with a population or comparing two samples with each other (e.g., a treatment vs. a control), the most typical procedure is the t-test. When comparing more than two groups (e.g., treatment 1, treatment 2, and treatment 3), we typically employ the F-test. The F-test uses the **analysis of variance (ANOVA)**. The F-test may also substitute for the t-test when comparing two groups, in which case $F = t^2$.

The ANOVA and its accompanying F-test offer a remarkably flexible family of techniques, used for the one-way design as well as the factorial designs described next. It can also provide a test for equivalence of variances (e.g., $\sigma_B^2 = \sigma_G^2$) and for significant increments in multiple regression (see the section "Multiple Regression" later in this chapter). Thus F-tests pop up in many research studies for a variety of purposes.

In the one-way and factorial designs, we analyze only one dependent variable at a time. For example, the dependent variable may consist of a score on a depression inventory. Hence we call these *univariate* designs. The prefix *uni-* refers to the number of dependent variables, namely, one—though we may have more than one independent variable, as in a factorial design.

Many studies have more than one dependent variable. For example, a psychotherapy outcome study may use scores on tests of depression, anxiety, therapeutic alliance, and treatment satisfaction. In such a study, the researcher may use four separate F-tests to analyze these four dependent variables.

However, the preferred procedure involves using *multivariate analysis of variance* (MANOVA), which analyzes all four dependent variables at once. In the process of doing so, MANOVA takes into account the degree of relationship among the dependent variables and helps to protect against the compounding of probabilities when conducting multiple tests (see earlier discussion of Type I error). Note that MANOVA deals with multiple dependent variables, whereas a factorial design deals with multiple independent variables. Researchers frequently use MANOVA with factorial designs when the study has multiple dependent variables as well as multiple independent variables.

A third type of test statistic is χ^2 (chi-square). The t- and F-test statistics apply most often when the dependent variable is measured on a continuous scale, as with the score on a depression inventory. The χ^2 statistic applies when data fall on a nominal scale, for example, classification of persons by a category such as gender (male or female) or diagnosis (e.g., anxiety disorder, mood disorder, or substance disorder). However, like the F-test, χ^2 is a remarkably flexible tool and pops up in a surprising array of applications. All three of the tests (t, F, and χ^2) use the mechanisms of NHST as described above.

Research Designs

A research study typically follows one of several basic designs. Each design has its strengths and weaknesses. In this section, we summarize the common designs and what to watch out for when evaluating a study using each. When first encountering a research study, identifying its basic design will help alert you to its shortcomings.

True Experimental Design

The "gold standard" for empirical research in behavioral health and addictions is the **true experimental design**. In clinical contexts, we call this design the **randomized clinical trial (RCT)** or randomized controlled trial. We must exercise care using the words *experiment* and *experimental*. In ordinary conversation, they can simply mean new or different. In the world of research, the term *experiment* has a much more specific meaning, as we describe here.

The true experimental design has five key features. Figure 5.2 illustrates these features for the two-group case, comparing a treatment group with a control group.

1. The design starts with a participant pool. The pool might contain, for example, all children identified with ADHD in a school system or all postmenopausal women self-referred to a particular clinic.

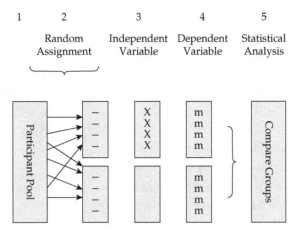

FIGURE 5.2 Key features of a randomized clinical trial for a two-group case.

2. The researcher assigns members of the participant pool at **random** to one of the groups, in this case to the treatment (experimental) group or to the control group. Random assignment is *essential* and constitutes the defining characteristic of the true experimental design. Common methods of random assignment to groups include using tables of random numbers, flipping a coin, or drawing names from a hat. Many software packages contain routines for drawing random numbers. Any nonrandom method of assignment destroys the experimental design. For example, placing all ADHD cases from one school building into the treatment group and cases from another school building into the control group is *not* random assignment. Placing the more severe cases of depression into the treatment group and using less severe cases as controls is *not* random assignment.

3. An **independent variable** is applied. In the clinical context, the independent variable usually consists of a treatment, for example, psychodynamic therapy or medication, versus no treatment. The experimental group receives the treatment and the control group does not. Or the design may involve two types of treatment, for example, a psychodynamic therapy for one group and pharmacotherapy for the other group. All circumstances other than the independent variable remain constant or vary at random between the two groups.

4. Following application of the independent variable, the research-ers measure the **dependent variable**. The dependent variable defines the behavior or outcome of interest in the research. It may consist of the score on a test, clinicians' judgment of improvement, clients' self-report of change, or some type of behavioral count. Typically, the design includes several depen-dent variables. For example, a study may include all four of the variables just mentioned: a test score, clinicians' judgment, patient self-report, and behavioral count.

5. Finally, the investigator applies statistical analysis to the depen-dent variable in order to compare the two groups. The result typically employs a **significance test,** such as a t-test, F-test, or chi-square (χ^2), accompanied by a declaration of whether the difference between the groups is statistically significant or nonsignificant and, preferably, a measure of effect size.

WHY IS IT THE GOLD STANDARD?

In EBP, multiple types of research designs are valued, but they are ranked according to a hierarchy of evidence. The hierarchy flows from the relative strength of each research design in providing results that prove valid and useful, especially in causally deter-mining therapeutic effects. Research methodologists use the term *internal validity* to characterize a study's basis for warranting a causal conclusion.

The hierarchy of evidence incorporates both research designs and the way in which the results of research get summarized. The APA (2005) policy on EBP, for example, states, "The validity of conclusions from research on interventions is based on a general progression from clinical observation through systematic reviews of randomized clinical trials."

At the top of the hierarchy sit meta-analyses and systematic reviews of RCTs. Meta-analyses and systematic reviews prefer RCTs but certainly do not limit their focus to that type of design. They include studies using other design types, as explained later in this chapter. For example, a meta-analysis may incorporate both RCTs and quasi-experimental studies or consist entirely of correlational studies.

Right below meta-analyses and reviews of RCTs on the hierar-chy of research evidence come individual RCTs, followed by cohort studies, which provide incidence, follow-up, and longitudinal data. On the bottom of the hierarchy sit case reports, clinical observations, and commentary. As we frequently hear in EBP circles, "the plural of anecdote is not research evidence."

Three crucial caveats accompany the established hierarchy. First, the "best" research design depends upon the specific clinical question. Randomized clinical trials prove practically meaningless for answering most epidemiological, diagnostic, and assessment questions.

Second, RCTs do not constitute the only sort of research evidence, merely the most preferred. Wholesale discounting of evidence from other research designs is unwarranted and contrary to EBP principles.

And third, not all important questions can or will be addressed by controlled research. This point was convincingly made in a spoof of the more radical evidence-based medicine articles (G. C. S. Smith & Pell, 2003). Unable to locate a single RCT on the use of parachutes, the authors (sarcastically) deplored their routine use. They condemned people for relying solely on observational data and using parachutes without controlled trials attesting to their efficacy!

Indeed, the greatest shortcoming of the RCT design is precisely that it cannot address many questions because we cannot use random assignment for many topics. For ethical reasons, physical reasons, or both, we cannot randomly assign people to their gender, their socioeconomic level, their degree of depression, their history of substance abuse, their age, and so on. Nor can we, on ethical grounds, randomly assign participants to all treatment alternatives or to those proven harmful; for instance, one cannot randomly assign patients to nonempathic, judgmental therapists versus empathic, supportive therapists or to unloving, disengaged parents versus loving, attached parents. For circumstances like these, we must rely on other types of research designs, all of which preclude drawing firm causal conclusions.

Most researchers consider the RCT the gold standard among research designs because it is the only one that allows for drawing a causal conclusion: that the variation in the independent variable causes the difference in the dependent variable. More specifically, the only possible differences between the groups result from (1) the independent variable and (2) random differences. The statistical test accounts for the random differences. If the difference between groups exceeds what we can attribute to random sampling variation, then the independent variable remains as the only possible explanation for the difference. In effect, the RCT allows us to make causal statements regarding the efficacy of the treatment, at least in the controlled context of the experiment.

RANDOM ASSIGNMENT VERSUS RANDOM SAMPLING

As noted above, random assignment of participants to the different groups or conditions is an essential feature of the RCT design. We must carefully distinguish between such random assignment and the notion of random sampling from a population.

Random sampling from a population underlies the model used in elementary statistical inference. We start with a well-defined population, for example, all children with ADHD or all men with cocaine dependence. Then we take a random sample from this population. Research studies rarely operate with this model because investigators seldom have access to large populations from which to easily conscript randomly selected participants. Rather, research studies usually start with some ad hoc or convenience group of individuals and then randomly assign the members of the group to conditions in the study. With random assignment to conditions, the true experimental design works.

However, that does not mean that the results will generalize to some well-defined population. In fact, this constitutes one of the major problems with research studies even when they do use random assignment. To what population do the results generalize? The answer usually becomes a judgment call not subject to careful statistical reasoning and procedures.

We must also distinguish between a random sample and a *representative* sample. A representative sample accurately reflects important characteristics of the population, where the meaning of "important" varies depending on the topic being studied. One can draw a simple random sample in such a way that each element of the population has an equal chance of entering into the sample. A random sample is *not* necessarily representative, as many people incorrectly suppose. Any particular random sample may prove quite unrepresentative of the larger population. The value of using a random sample lies in the fact that rules of probability define the likelihood that the random sample will prove representative.

Factorial Designs

The RCT typically has one independent variable and we therefore sometimes call it a one-way design. A factorial design has more than one independent variable operating at the same time. For example, one independent variable may be the type of treatment (control, medication, or integrative therapy) and the other may involve duration of the intervention (6 weeks or 12 weeks). Figure 5.3 outlines this design. Participants are assigned at random to each of the cells in this design. Each *m* is a measure on a participant in the study, say, a measure of self-reported improvement.

The factorial design allows for analyzing the effect of type of treatment and the effect of length of treatment (time) within the same study. We call the separate effect of each of these variables a **main effect** in the study. The unique feature of the factorial design is that it allows for the study of possible **interaction** between independent variables. An interaction might occur if the effectiveness of the type of treatment differed depending on the length of treatment. We designate this interaction as "treatment × time," read as "treatment by time." We can identify such interactions only if we use a factorial design. Hence, such designs provide a powerful addition to the researcher's toolkit.

Simply identifying that an interaction is significant does not reveal the nature of that interaction. Understanding an interaction in a factorial design requires examination of cell means (i.e., the mean for all cases within each cell). A graph of the cell means then tells the story of the interaction. Figure 5.4 shows the cell means for

	Treatment		
Time	Control	Medication	Therapy
6 wks	m m m m m m m m	m m m m m m m m	m m m m m m m m
12 wks	m m m m m m m m	m m m m m m m m	m m m m m m m m

FIGURE 5.3 An example of a 3 × 2 factorial design.

		Treatment	
Time	Control	Medication	Therapy
6 wks	10	20	15
12 wks	12	14	22

FIGURE 5.4 Cell means in a 3 × 2 factorial design.

the treatment × time design in Figure 5.3, and Figure 5.5 shows the plot of the cell means. We have used self-reported improvement, on which we consider a high score favorable, as the outcome measure (dependent variable).

In this case, the plot shows that the medication is more effective than the integrative therapy at the 6-week duration but that integrative therapy becomes more effective than the medication at the 12-week duration.

We have described a two-way factorial design above. We might have more than two independent variables, resulting in a three-way or four-way design. In fact, the number of independent variables has no limit, although we rarely encounter more than three in any one study. Many variations on the assignment of participants in factorial designs also exist.

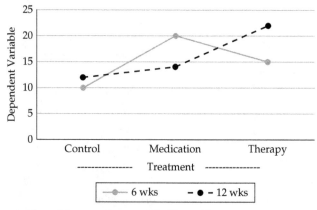

FIGURE 5.5 Plot of interaction revealed by cell means.

In the example just given, both independent variables were true, manipulated variables. Hence, we can draw causal conclusions about both of them. We often find that in a factorial design one or more (even all) variables are natural group variables, such as gender or age (see later discussion of natural group contrasts under "Quasi-experimental Designs"). When that occurs, we cannot draw causal conclusions about the natural group variable(s). For example, in Figure 5.3, substitute gender (men vs. women) for the time variable (6 weeks vs. 12 weeks). Gender qualifies as a natural group variable. We do not assign cases at random to gender categories. Thus, use of a factorial design does not automatically mean that the design qualifies as a true experimental design. We must examine the nature of the independent variables and the method of assigning cases to groups to determine whether we can draw causal conclusions.

Quasi-experimental Designs

Quasi-experimental designs comprise a whole family of research designs, all of which try to approximate the RCT. Crucially, however, none of the quasi-experimental designs features random assignment.

NATURAL GROUP CONTRASTS

Quasi-experimental designs fall into three broad categories. The first category involves *natural group contrasts*. For example, we may compare children with and without ADHD or severely and moderately depressed women. The natural group contrast easily extends to comparisons among more than two groups, for example, nondepressed, moderately depressed, and severely depressed women. Such natural group contrasts look very much like experimental designs.

Figure 5.6 outlines a natural group contrast study. Notice how similar it seems to the true experimental design in Figure 5.2. Both designs have contrasting groups, an independent variable, and a dependent variable. The statistical analysis proceeds in *exactly* the same manner whether the design follows an experimental or a quasi-experimental model. The difference involves the random assignment of participants to conditions in the experimental design but not in the quasi-experimental design. Natural groups in the quasi-experimental

Natural Groups	Independent Variable	Dependent Variable	Statistical Analysis

FIGURE 5.6 The common natural group contrast quasi-experimental design.

design may (and probably do) differ in numerous ways in addition to the nominal basis for their grouping.

For example, consider the nominal classification of gender: men and women. Subjects likely differ not only in gender but also in average height, arm strength, interests, socialization, hormonal levels, and numerous other variables. Thus, if we find a difference in the dependent variable between men and women, it may, at the root, result from a difference between people of different heights or some other variable rather than from the difference in gender. We call these other variables **confounds**. They become confounded or mixed up with the nominal basis for classification and literally confound our interpretation of results from natural group contrasts.

Research often involves natural group contrasts that yield results subject to misinterpretation. People seem to have an irresistible urge to attribute causality to the nominal basis for the classification without taking into account the many confounding variables.

TIME SERIES DESIGNS

A second broad category in the quasi-experimental family involves *time series*. The simplest case is an off–on (or AB) design. We measure a group of participants for, say, alcohol abuse before the introduction of an independent variable (treatment). This is the off condition. Then the treatment switches "on" and we again measure participants' alcohol abuse. If alcohol abuse decreases, one could reason that the treatment worked. The design is weak in that a host of factors might have affected the participants in addition to the treatment, including the fact that we monitored their alcohol abuse twice. Thus, a strengthened design would flow as off–on–off–on–off–on (or ABABAB). Many variations of time series designs exist, but all attempt to find the elusive causal connection between independent and dependent variables. All suffer from lack of random assignment.

ANALYSIS OF COVARIANCE

A third broad category of quasi-experimental designs involves techniques that rely strictly on statistical analysis. The most common of these, **analysis of covariance (ANCOVA)**, focuses on adjusting the results of the comparison between groups on the dependent variable for possible differences in confounding variables. These analyses give rise to conclusions such as "the groups differed in ability even after accounting for differences in socioeconomic level" or "the groups differed in levels of depression even after equating them on anxiety." Such expressions signal the use of ANCOVA.

However, one never knows whether another confounding variable might still be operating. The independent variable of interest (say, a psychotherapy) may become confounded with a host of other variables. For example, using the natural groups contrast, we might compare outcomes for a group of ADHD boys receiving a behavioral treatment at Lincoln School with a group of ADHD boys not receiving the treatment at Washington School. We determine that the outcomes are favorable for the boys receiving the treatment in comparison with those not receiving the treatment. We would like to conclude that the treatment proved effective. But we remain stuck with the possibility that many other differences exist between the two groups besides the treatment variable. Perhaps Lincoln School has facilities or teachers that make it a nicer place. Perhaps one of the schools recently changed principals. Perhaps the root of the differences in outcomes lies in the neighborhoods the two schools serve. We can make the same type of argument for any of the quasi-experimental designs. Even when ANCOVA "equates" the groups on some extraneous variables, the possibility always exists that some other variable, not captured in the covariance, influenced the outcome.

Identifying Causal Words

A truism of research design holds that one cannot draw causal conclusions from any quasi-experimental design. When examining quasi-experimental research, remain alert to inappropriate use of the words *cause* and *causal*. However, the English language contains many words that imply causation, and you should be equally alert to inappropriate use of such words. Here we provide a partial list of such words, where the words on the left suggest a positive causal impact and the words on the right suggest a negative causal impact:

Leads to	Undermines
Produces	Reduces
Increases	Decreases
Raises	Lowers
Enhances	Undercuts
Improves	Damages
Boosts	Eases
Develops	Weakens

Beware of any of these terms suggesting a causal link. They apply appropriately only when the research design is adequate to the task. Inappropriate use of such words in the context of nonexperimental designs plagues even the professional literature.

As well, beware the term *predict* in clinical reports. Saying that "family conflict predicts substance abuse" only means that the two variables are correlated, not that one early in life causes the other later in life. To a clinician and layperson, *predict* often implies longitudinal causality; however, to a researcher, it does not. So unless the study involved a 20-year longitudinal data collection, beware the use of *predict*.

Survey Designs

Mental health and addiction research makes wide use of surveys. Such surveys comprise the principal source of information about prevalence rates (see "Prevalence Rates and Related Ratios" in Chapter 6). We also use surveys routinely to solicit people's reactions to policies, practices, programs, and procedures. A survey design includes the population we want to sample, the method of participant selection, the method of contact, the survey questions, and the method of analysis and reporting.

An important matter in sampling from a population concerns the definition of the *sampling frame*. The sampling frame lists specific elements in the population and becomes the operational definition of the population. We need to stay alert to possible mismatch between the sampling frame and the population of real interest. For example, a population of interest may be the residents of a particular city, and the sampling frame may focus on the telephone directory for that city. However, some residents of the city do not have a telephone, have unlisted numbers, or use only a cell phone. Other residents of the city have more than one entry in the telephone directory. Thus the sampling frame in this instance does not align perfectly with the population of interest.

Some surveys do not involve sampling from a population. Rather, an entire group, albeit a small one, forms the desired respondent group. For example, we may aim a survey at all 300 persons currently under care in a psychiatric hospital or all adolescents attending a partial hospitalization program, where these groups precisely represent our interest. In such cases, methods of sampling become irrelevant and we do not need inferential statistics (e.g., standard errors).

Another important consideration for survey designs involves sample size. Surveys usually report the *margin of error* for the results. In the language of survey methods, confidence intervals defined by the standard error of a percentage (SE_p) constitute the survey's margin of error—percentage being the most common metric used for reporting survey results. Thus a report may say, "The margin of error for the survey was ±3 points." Sample size (N) enters into the equation for this standard error.

 The book's companion website contains a file that shows standard errors of percentage for simple random samples, translated into confidence intervals, for a response percentage of 50% (e.g., 50% "Yes" answers on a survey question) at different levels of N from 10 to 1,000. You can enter any value for N and see the resulting confidence intervals. Note the effect of the sample size on the confidence intervals.

Another crucial aspect of any survey concerns the nonresponse rate. Many surveys have substantial nonresponse rates. When this occurs, the nonresponse rate creates a far greater potential source of error than the official margin of error. Suppose the target sample contains 500 people, of whom 40% (200) respond and 60% (300) do not respond. Among respondents, 75% answer "Yes" to a certain question. Theoretically, anywhere from 0 to 300 of the nonrespondents might have answered "Yes" to this question. Hence, the final percentage answering "Yes" could range anywhere from 30% to 90%. The margin of error based on nonresponse in this example is 60%, whereas the "official" margin of error based solely on the respondent group is only 6% (a 95% confidence interval). Reporting a margin of error at only 6% would grossly mislead readers. The best one can hope for in such circumstances would be for the researchers to demonstrate that the nonrespondent group presented as highly similar to the respondent group on a host of variables relevant to the survey topics.

A final source of difficulty for interpretation of survey results is the manner in which the investigator summarizes results. A simple example makes the point. Take this question: "Do you think your treatment was effective?" The responses compute as follows: yes, 45%; no, 25%; unsure, 30%. This array of responses supports all of the following assertions, which give different impressions of the results: (a) Only a minority of respondents believed the treatment was effective. (b) Only a minority of the respondents believed the treatment was ineffective. (c) Of those who reached a conclusion about the treatment, a majority believed the treatment was effective. Our point: Examine actual response data to interpret conclusions. (Note that this matter of how the data are summarized stands quite apart from the problem of how the survey questions are worded.)

Observational Studies

Observational studies concentrate on obtaining an accurate description of some phenomenon. They may attempt to provide an overall description, for example, by observing and describing what Jonathon, our 8-year-old ADHD patient, does during a 1-hour period in his classroom. Or they may focus on observations concentrated on a specific, operationalized behavior. For example, again for Jonathon, how frequently does he engage in off-task behavior during a 5-minute period? Investigators often report results from such focused observations in the form of counts or checklists.

All scientific investigations begin with observations; observations form the original "stuff" of science. However, observational studies result chiefly in descriptions. They lack explanatory power. They may suggest avenues for later work leading to explanations, but they do not themselves provide explanations and causal connections. As a consequence, we rarely see them considered in evidence-based compilations.

Case Studies

The **case study method** involves detailed descriptions of individual cases or of small numbers of similar cases. Some case studies limit themselves to pure description, but researchers often attempt to suggest causes of behavior(s) manifest in the cases. The case study method can prove particularly valuable when we are attempting to understand new or rare conditions for which insufficient numbers of cases exist to allow any other type of study. The case study method does not permit drawing strong conclusions, simply because it involves only one or a few cases. Causal connections suggested in well-written, highly detailed case studies, such as those by Freud, can sound persuasive, so one must exercise caution in drawing conclusions from such reports.

Multivariate Techniques

Behavioral health and addiction research has become replete with reports using multivariate statistics. However, the typical report using one of these techniques relies on a few basic mechanisms, summarized below to enhance your interpretation and application of such studies.

Partial Correlation

To begin, consider this important point about partial correlations: We do not find them reported frequently in the research literature.

However, they underlie much of the work carried out with other multivariate techniques. Thus, gaining some familiarity with this topic will prove critical in understanding what happens with other multivariate techniques.

Partial correlation is a procedure for expressing the degree of relationship between two variables (A and B) with a third variable (C) "held constant" or "partialed out." We accomplish the holding constant by predicting A and B from C. Figure 5.7 shows the sequence of steps involved in determining the partial correlation coefficient of variables A and B with C partialed out. We express the result as $r_{AB.C}$, read as "the correlation between A and B with C held constant [or partialed out]." We also say we have "removed the effect of C."

Consider this example. In a group of children aged 8–13 years, we find the following correlations among chronological age (C), mental age (M), and shoe size (S):

$$r_{CM} = .65 \quad r_{CS} = .75 \quad r_{MS} = .50$$

What happens to the correlation between mental age and shoe size when age is held constant? The partial correlation $r_{MS.C}$ is .02. Hence, with chronological age held constant, the correlation between mental age and shoe size, originally .50, approximates 0!

 The book's companion website provides a worksheet with sample values used to calculate partial r. You can substitute other values to explore the effect of partialing out a third variable.

We can sometimes hold a third variable constant by the way we collect data. In the example just discussed, we could accomplish this by collecting data only on children within a 1-year age span, say, only children 8 years old. However, frequently it will prove inconvenient or impossible to hold a third variable constant in the data collection stage. Partial correlation proves particularly useful in those circumstances.

Note that we can hold constant or partial out more than one variable. In fact, researchers frequently do so. For example, $r_{AB.CDE}$

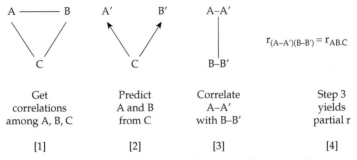

FIGURE 5.7 Sequence of steps for partialing out a third variable.

indicates the correlation between *A* and *B* with *C, D,* and *E* partialed out or held constant.

Multiple Regression

Multiple regression is a set of techniques for expressing the relationship between one variable (the *criterion*) and a composite of other variables, with the composite constructed so as to apply optimal weights to each entry. "Optimal" weights are those that maximize the relationship between the criterion and the composite of predictor variables. For example, we may predict suicidal ideation (the criterion) from three predictors: level of depression, self-reported quality of life, and age.

A multiple regression provides a correlation between the criterion and the composite. We call this a *multiple correlation*, designated by *R*. Subscripts on *R* indicate the predicted variable and which variables fall in the composite of predictors. For example, the designation $R_{Y.123}$ indicates the multiple correlation of *Y* (the criterion) with the optimal composite of variables 1, 2, and 3.

An outcome of a multiple regression analysis is a multiple regression equation. Research reports often present this equation. It may look like this: $Y = b_1X_1 + b_2X_2 + b_3X_3 + c$, where b_i is the weight given to each predictor X_i. In some versions, *b* appears as the Greek letter beta (β). The beta weights help us understand the contribution each variable makes to the prediction.

Perhaps the most crucial point to consider about the weights applied in the regression equation is this: They depend not only on the correlation of each predictor variable with the criterion but also on the correlations among the predictors. A predictor may have a reasonably high correlation with the criterion, but if it also has a high correlation with other predictors, then it will not receive a large weight and in fact may be eliminated from the equation completely. For instance, in our example of suicidal ideation, we may begin a prediction model with four tests covering depression, anxiety, self-efficacy, and negative affect. All correlate substantially with suicide ideation. However, negative affect and depression may correlate so highly with one another that one will drop out of the prediction equation—with no loss in predictive power. Partial correlations play the key role in sorting through this complex of relationships.

A common analysis developed from a multiple regression involves examining the increase in R as we add different variables to or delete them from the regression equation. This type of analysis introduces the terms R^2 and ΔR^2 (read "delta R-squared"). The delta represents the *difference* (increase or decrease) in R^2 as we add or remove variables. Does adding a variable to the equation significantly increase R^2? To follow our example from above, would adding a measure of hopelessness significantly improve our prediction of suicidal ideation? If it does, we want to add that variable to the equation. If adding the variable to the equation does not significantly increase R^2 (i.e., if ΔR^2 is small), then we have no good reason to add the variable. Similarly, we can ask whether deleting a variable leads to little change in R^2. If so, we can eliminate the variable with no significant loss in predictive power.

A researcher has several options for conducting a multiple regression analysis. The options relate to such matters as the method for entering variables into the analysis and rules for when to stop entering or removing variables. However, all of the points made above apply to interpreting results regardless of the options chosen by the researcher.

Logistic Regression

Logistic regression has similarities to multiple regression in that it aims to predict one variable (the criterion) from an optimal combination of several other variables. Logistic regression differs from multiple regression mainly in the nature of the variables involved in the analysis. Most typically in multiple regression we focus only on continuous variables. In logistic regression, criterion variables usually take dichotomous form, and at least some of the predictor variables are discrete. Examples of dichotomous variables are ADHD/non-ADHD, depressed/not depressed, and dead/alive. We might use logistic regression to predict membership in the ADHD group from gender, score above a cut point on an ADHD scale, and teacher nomination. The logistic regression provides the optimal weighting of these three predictor variables to predict membership in the ADHD group (or, conversely, in the non-ADHD group). It is possible to have discrete categories with more than two groups (e.g., severely depressed, mildly depressed, and not depressed), but these categories get converted into sets of dichotomies in the analysis.

Because of the dichotomous criterion variable in logistic regression, researchers will generally interpret the final result of the analysis as a probability or some transformation of a probability. For example, given a set of predictor variables with their optimal weights, what is the probability that a child belongs to the ADHD group? A common transformation of the probability from logistic regression is the **odds ratio** (see "Odds Ratio and Relative Risk" in Chapter 6). Two statistical procedures similar to logistic regression in their purpose and in at least some of their procedures are discriminant analysis and cluster analysis. However, we do not see these analyses used as much as logistic regression in behavioral health research.

Factor Analysis

Factor analysis is a family of data reduction techniques designed to identify basic dimensions (*factors*) among a multiplicity of variables. We start with many specific items, for example, scores on 20 personality measures, and then determine the correlations among these measures. Factor analytic techniques operate with these correlations. As variables we may use scores on entire tests or single items within tests.

The reasoning, which actually operates in the form of mathematical functions, proceeds as follows. If we find that two variables correlate very highly (say, $r = .90$), we can think of these two variables as if they fall along a single dimension. Similarly, say that four of the original variables correlated highly with one another; we could then collapse these four variables into a single dimension or factor. We cannot collapse variables that do not correlate highly. Factor analysis techniques analyze all the relationships among the original variables to determine how many factors are needed to account for the relationships.

Research reports tend to concentrate on four outcomes of factor analysis:

◆ the factor matrix,
◆ the percentages of variance accounted for by factors,
◆ rules for when to stop extracting factors, and
◆ the naming of the factors.

Figure 5.8 presents an example of a factor matrix. In this case, the factor analysis yields four factors for the 15 items using one of the standard criteria for extracting factors. We call entries in the body of the table loadings. They express the relationship between each theoretical factor and each item. Loadings of .40 or higher are shown in bold. By custom, although it is not mandatory, we highlight high loadings (say, over .30 or over .40) with bold, italics, or underlining. These highlighted items best represent the apparent underlying dimension. Entries below the table show the percentage of the total variance for the 15 items accounted for by each factor and the percentage of the variance covered by the four factors accounted for by each factor.

As you read a research report, stay alert to when the researchers stopped extracting factors. The mathematical routines for factor analysis will continue to extract factors up to the limit of the number of variables in the analysis. However, factors extracted later in the process will often prove meaningless, because they account for so little variance. A research report will usually identify the criterion used for stopping the extraction process, and ordinarily one can accept the researchers' choice of criterion.

The analysis displayed in Figure 5.8 shows one dominant factor accounting for over half of the variance covered by the four factors, although covering somewhat less than one third of the total variance. Then we have three weaker factors, with the fourth one of marginal utility. Naming the factors calls for judgment and insight rather than a mechanical or mathematical process. One examines the variables with highest loadings on each factor to see what they seem to have in common and then develops a word or a few words that capture the essence of the factor.

What we just described is called *exploratory factor analysis* (EFA): It explores the underlying factor structure. **Confirmatory**

Item	Factor			
	1	2	3	4
1	−.006	**.439**	.177	**.737**
2	.073	.343	−.038	.035
3	.177	.097	**.644**	.183
4	.113	.092	.747	.188
5	**.467**	.193	.240	−.006
6	.393	.328	**.426**	−.042
7	.156	−.149	.216	**.431**
8	**.442**	.006	.215	.099
9	**.755**	.139	.016	.101
10	**.809**	.099	.035	.133
11	.307	**.583**	.202	−.091
12	.371	**.504**	.319	.165
13	**.678**	.293	.226	−.047
14	.311	.295	.085	−.012
15	.031	**.597**	.109	.053
Percent of total variance accounted for	31	10	10	7
Percent of variance accounted for by the 4 factors	53	17	17	12

FIGURE 5.8 Example of factor analysis results.

factor analysis (CFA), by contrast, begins with a theory about the underlying factor structure and then attempts to show that the factor data fit the theory. For example, we may hypothesize that the correlations among the Wechsler intelligence subtests best fit a four-factor model. We use CFA to test the fit of this model. Confirmatory factor analysis is a type of structural equation modeling, so we delay describing it further until our next section.

Structural Equation Modeling

Structural equation modeling (SEM) attempts to infer causal connections among many interrelated variables. Structural equation modeling starts with correlations among the variables. (Actually, most work with SEM uses the covariance matrix, but we refer to cor-relations here because they are the more familiar metric.) As every statistics textbook emphasizes, one cannot infer causation from cor-relation coefficients. The modeling techniques suspend this truism. Essentially, they say: Let us suppose that causal connections do exist among these intercorrelated variables and that we can surmise the directions of these connections based on theory or research to build a model showing the causal relationships among the variables.

As with all multivariate techniques, SEM, sometimes called *causal modeling* precisely because it imputes causality, includes a variety of specific approaches. One example is *path analysis*, aptly named because it shows paths (with causal directions) among a number of variables.

The most distinctive feature of a structural equation model is the diagram showing the relationships and causal directions among variables. The presence of such a diagram signals that the investiga-tor has used SEM. Text accompanying the diagram provides verbal descriptions of relationships depicted in the diagram.

Figure 5.9 shows a simplified path model (adapted from Holahan et al., 2005). The model attempts to "explain" 10-Year Depressive Symptoms (on the far right in the figure). Single-headed arrows show implied causal direction. The double-headed arrow between Baseline Avoidance Coping and Baseline Depressive Symptoms shows that they mutually influence each other. Baseline Avoidance Coping directly influences status on 4-Year Life Stressors. Notice that in this model, Baseline Avoidance Coping does not influence 10-Year Depressive Symptoms directly; rather, 4-Year Life Stressors *mediates* the influence of Baseline Avoidance Coping on 10-Year

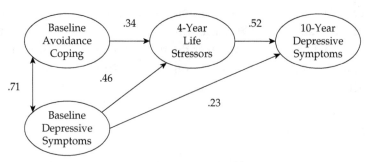

FIGURE 5.9 Example of a path model. Adapted from Holahan et al. (2005).

Depressive Symptoms. (See "Mediation Analysis" later in this chapter.) In contrast, Baseline Depressive Symptoms has a direct influence on 10-Year Depressive Symptoms as well as indirect effects through both 4-Year Life Stressors and the influence of Baseline Depressive Symptoms on 4-Year Life Stressors. Coefficients on each arrow indicate the strength of the relationship.

A structural equation model begins its analysis with a correlation matrix (or covariance matrix). It then applies multiple regression and partial correlation procedures to the many possible relationships among the variables; it may also use factor analysis to form composite variables, often called *latent variables*.

Most importantly, before the analysis begins, the researcher must have a theory about the causal connections among the variables. This theory guides the specific analyses used to trace paths through the network of relationships. Customarily some measure of "fit" tells how well the theoretical model agrees with the actual data, that is, the original set of correlations. Typically, two or more models will be "fit" to the data, and the researcher hopes to show that the proposed model provides the best fit. One must remember that the model, no matter how good the fit, flows from correlations that do not themselves point in causal directions. (For more on SEM, see Kline, 2011, and Schumacker & Lomax, 2016).

 Skill Exercise 5-4

Structural equation models can become exceedingly complex. To become familiar with their representation, enter "images of structural equation models" into any Internet search engine. You will see many models, most having links to their original articles or other sources. Click on an image, then on the button for "view page."

We return now to the topic of confirmatory factor analysis (CFA) which, as noted above, is a subcategory of structural equation modeling. Figure 5.10 illustrates a typical application for CFA, using concepts and procedures from SEM. The question we want the analysis to address is how best to conceptualize the psychological construct "self-confidence." In the language of SEM, self-confidence constitutes

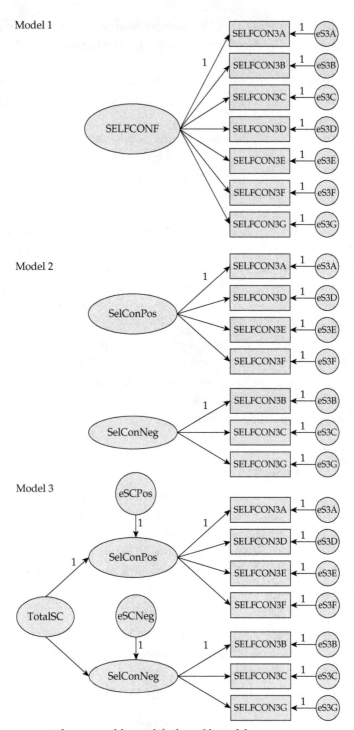

FIGURE 5.10 Three possible models for self-confidence.

a latent variable. The concept is the same as a factor in factor analysis or a construct in psychological assessment. Latent variables typically get represented as ovals in SEM. We have seven measures of self-confidence; actual measures (data or observed variables) typically get represented as rectangles in SEM.

For our seven measures, is it best to conceptualize self-confidence by model 1, 2, or 3? Model 1 says self-confidence is a single latent variable. Model 2 says, no, it is not a single variable but rather two variables—a positive aspect to self-confidence and a negative aspect to self-confidence—and they act independently of each other. Model 3 says, well, you are both partly right: There are two separate aspects to self-confidence, but they can accumulate into a total. One can easily imagine parallel questions' being raised about the structure of intelligence, subjective well-being, and a host of other psychological constructs.

Now we ask, which model best fits the data? (We have not described the data here, but think of it as the responses of 600 grade-4 students on the seven measures of self-confidence, converted into a covariance matrix.) The procedures of SEM (and CFA) fit the data to the models (or the models to the data), yielding several *fit statistics* to help answer the question of which fit works best. Books on SEM give guidelines for what is acceptable fit and whether one fit differs materially from another fit. The important point for EBP is understanding how these procedures help us to think about the underlying variables (or constructs, dimensions, factors) we deal with when interacting with patients.

Mediation Analysis

The **mediator** is an important concept in behavioral science, indeed in all of science. When two variables are related, what really lies at the root of the relationship? We call the process of sorting through this issue *mediation analysis,* and it is intimately connected with notions of SEM. We present here a simple model of mediation analysis. The classic mediation model proceeds through these steps:

1. *Start*: The variables X and Y are related (correlated). Invoke the "old saw" from Stat 101: Correlation does not imply causation.

Could be *X* influencing *Y*, could be *Y* influencing *X*, could be some other variable(s) influencing both *X* and *Y*.

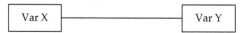

2. *Theorize:* Based on theory or other research, suspend the "old saw" and assert that the causal direction is from *X* to *Y*.

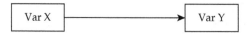

3. *Introduce mediator:* Based on further theory or research, assert that *X*'s influence on *Y* is not direct but is transmitted, at least in part, through a third variable *M*: the mediator.

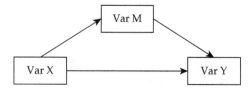

4. *Test for mediator's influence:* Apply mediation analytic techniques to determine how much of the *X–Y* relationship might be mediated through *M*. That is, what's left of the direct *X–Y* relationship after accounting for the role of the mediator? (This question is indicated by the question mark in the next diagram.) If the relationship of *X* to *Y* drops to zero, mediation is complete. If the relationship of *X* to *Y* decreases (but not to zero), mediation is partial. If the relationship of *X* to *Y* remains unchanged, there is no mediating influence of *M*.

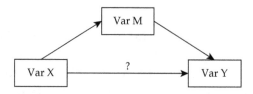

Consider the following example, which applies the steps just listed to a hypothetical study. We find a robust correlation between depression (*X*) and suicidal ideation (*Y*). Following the old saw in Step 1, depression may cause suicidal ideation, or suicidal ideation may cause depression. However, we assert or assume (Step 2) that causality flows from depression to suicidal ideation. Upon further reflection

(Step 3), we assume that depression influences *future concerns*—a mediating variable (*M*)—and that this variable influences suicidal ideation. We perform the mediation analysis (Step 4) and find that, indeed, the correlation between depression and suicidal ideation decreases substantially when we take into account future concerns. Thus, future concerns mediate the relationship between depression and suicidal ideation.

Remember these important points when examining and applying a mediation model:

◆ You can have more than one mediator. In fact, models can become quite complex, involving numerous mediators. (In the simple example presented here, we assumed only three variables operating.)
◆ We need to worry about the measurement reliability of all the variables.
◆ The mediator may significantly reduce an *X–Y* relationship, but you still have to determine the real-world strength of the mediator.
◆ Despite the highfalutin statistics, it's all still correlational.

 Skill Exercise 5-5

For a wealth of information about the concept of mediation, examples, and analytic techniques, visit David Kenny's mediation website: davidakenny.net/cm/mediate.htm

Summary Points About Multivariate Techniques

For all of the multivariate techniques, remember these key points: First, if the variables entering the multivariate analysis do not represent relevant or important facets of the clinical subject, the multivariate technique will not and cannot identify those facets. Multivariate analysis can only reveal relationships among the entered variables; it cannot tell us what is missing or what may be more important than the variables entered. For example, if you omit anxiety measures in a study, then you will not get an anxiety factor in your factor analysis. If no information about genetics or family history enters your structural equation model attempting to predict depression, then family genetics will not show up as an important mediator. Whenever interpreting results of multivariate analyses, always ask yourself this question: What important information might be missing from the mix?

Second, remember that multivariate techniques (except when applied in the context of an RCT) deal with correlations. Bear in mind the old saw that you can't infer causation from correlation. Thus, beware of causal language accompanying the results. Causality may be there—or it may not be, or it may be in a different direction.

Third, fit statistics do not tell the whole story. A model may fit well but still explain very little of the entire phenomenon. Be sure to keep in mind the big picture: the effect sizes (see Chapter 6).

Finally, multivariate techniques can confer an aura of supersophistication on a study. Remember that they are subject to the same limitations as other research techniques: adequacy of sample size, representativeness of samples, reliability and validity of measures, and some notion of effect size.

Concluding Comment

This chapter has highlighted essential features of research designs frequently used in behavioral health and addiction research. It serves as a primer, not a graduate-level statistics and research design course. Most of the research falls into recognizably distinct categories. Each category has its special strengths and weaknesses. Spotting the basic design used in a study and being alert to its strengths and weaknesses should help you to leverage the research literature effectively to inform your evidence-based practice.

Key Terms

alpha level (α)
analysis of covariance
  (ANCOVA)
analysis of variance (ANOVA)
Bonferroni correction
case study method
confidence interval

confirmatory factor
  analysis (CFA)
confound
dependent variable
effect size
factor analysis
independent variable

interaction
logistic regression
main effect
mediator
multiple regression
null hypothesis
null hypothesis significance
test (NHST)
odds ratio
partial correlation
power

random
randomized clinical trial (RCT)
research hypothesis
significance level
significance test
standard error of a statistic
statistical hypothesis
true experimental design
Type I error
Type II error

Recommended Readings and Websites

Brown, T. A. (2015). *Confirmatory factor analysis for applied research* (2nd ed.). New York, NY: Guilford.

Cohen, J. (1988). *Statistical power analysis for the behavioral sciences* (2nd ed.). Hillsdale, NJ: Erlbaum.

Cohen, J., Cohen, P., West, S. G., & Aiken, L. S. (2003). *Applied multiple regression/correlation analysis for the behavioral sciences* (3rd ed.). Mahwah, NJ: Erlbaum.

Division of Biostatistics, Department of Epidemiology and Biostatistics, School of Medicine, University of California, San Francisco (2006). Power and sample size programs. www.biostat.ucsf.edu/sampsize.html

Hayes, A. F. (2013). *Introduction to mediation, moderation, and conditional process analysis: A regression-based approach.* New York, NY: Guilford.

Hosmer, D. W., Jr., Lemeshow, S., & Sturdivant, R. X. (2013). *Applied logistic regression* (3rd ed.). Hoboken, NJ: Wiley.

Kirk, R. E. (2013). *Experimental design: Procedures for the behavioral sciences* (4th ed.). Thousand Oaks, CA: Sage.

Kenny, D. A. (2015). Mediate [Website on mediation analysis]. davidakenny.net/cm/mediate.htm

Schumacker, R. E., & Lomax, R. G. (2016). *A beginner's guide to structural equation modeling* (4th ed.). New York, NY: Routledge.

Tabachnick, B. G., & Fidell, L. S. (2013). *Using multivariate statistics* (6th ed.). Boston, MA: Pearson.

6

Reading and Interpreting the Research: Numbers and Measures

Nᴏᴛ ꜱᴜʀᴘʀɪꜱɪɴɢʟʏ, ᴛʜᴇ ʀᴇꜱᴇᴀʀᴄʜ ᴛʜᴀᴛ ꜰᴜᴇʟꜱ evidence-based practice (EBP) abounds with numbers. To make sense of and apply the research, you will need a degree of familiarity with the numbers most frequently employed. This chapter covers these frequently used numbers, defining each and giving examples typical of those encountered in behavioral health and addictions research. We have made a judicious selection from among the plethora of choices, based primarily on frequency of usage and utility in informing clinical practice.

The Normal Curve

Research literature often refers to the "normal curve," "assumptions of normality," "departures from normality," and "common benchmarks within the normal curve" such as z-scores and cutoff points. Figure 6.1 presents a graph of the normal curve. Reference points within the curve shown on the bottom include z-scores, percentiles,

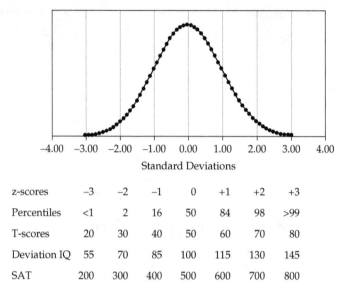

z-scores	−3	−2	−1	0	+1	+2	+3
Percentiles	<1	2	16	50	84	98	>99
T-scores	20	30	40	50	60	70	80
Deviation IQ	55	70	85	100	115	130	145
SAT		200	300	400	500	600	700	800

FIGURE 6.1 The normal curve and selected reference points.

T-scores, deviation IQs, and the familiar SAT score scale. Each of the last three reference systems uses a standard score, with means and standard deviations (SDs) of 50 and 10, 100 and 15, and 500 and 100, respectively.

We refer to the theoretical normal curve as *unimodal*—it has one "hump," reaching its maximum at the center of the distribution. The curve flows in a symmetrical shape about its center. At that center lie the mean, the median, and the mode. The tails of the distribution flow in an asymptotic manner with respect to the baseline (i.e., they approach the baseline but never touch it). Of course, in any actual distribution, the data set does have finite limits. The theoretical normal curve also has a certain relationship between its height and width. We might describe this characteristic as the curve's "shoulder" width, formally known as *kurtosis*.

Common departures from normality refer to the characteristics of *modality* and *symmetry*. Some distributions have more than one mode (hump); for example, a bimodal distribution has two humps. This happens rarely in behavioral health data. Many people assume that a bimodal distribution will result if we combine two distributions with different means (e.g., the heights of adult males and females). However, the two means must differ by at least 2 *SD*s for bimodality to result (Schilling et al., 2002). Two *SD*s represents a whopping big difference: Consider that mean heights for adult males and females—a very noticeable difference in daily life—differ by less than 2 *SD*s.

We call departures from the symmetry of the normal curve *skewness*. When data pile up at the low end of the curve, with a long tail to the right, we have *positive skewness* or *skewness to the right*. We refer to piling up at the high end with a long tail to the left as *negative skewness* or *skewness to the left*. Many distributions in the behavioral sciences exhibit abnormal skewness in one direction or the other, sometimes wreaking havoc with assumptions made in statistical analyses.

Confidence Intervals and Standard Errors

In behavioral health and addiction research, we often refer to *confidence intervals* and *standard errors*, which are intimately related. Two main types of standard errors and resulting confidence intervals demand our attention: those for test scores and those for statistics. Although the terms used for these two types seem similar, they refer to two quite different issues. We take them up in turn.

Confidence Interval for a Test Score

Construction of a **confidence interval (CI)** for a test score depends on reliability within the context of classical test theory, and specifically the notions of obtained score, true score, and error score. An **obtained score** indicates what we actually get for an individual on one occasion. The person's **true score** represents what we really want to know—but never have. We can think of it as the score a person would receive if we had a perfectly reliable test (i.e., a test with a standard error of zero). Alternatively, we may think of the true score as the average of an infinite number of obtained scores for an individual (assuming no fatigue from taking an infinite number of tests, no recollection of content from earlier administrations, and so on). The **error score** is the difference between the true score and the obtained score.

We commonly represent the relationship among the three as

$$O = T \pm E \quad \text{or} \quad T = O \pm E$$

where T represents the true score, O the obtained score, and E the error score. Thus the obtained score equals the true score plus or minus error due to unreliability. Conversely, the true score would equal the obtained score contaminated by unreliable error.

We assume that if we had an infinite number of obtained scores, the obtained scores would distribute themselves normally around the true score, which equals the mean or expected value for the entire distribution. Figure 6.2 illustrates this theoretical distribution of many obtained scores around a true score. Of course, we never get an infinite number of obtained scores. We get just one obtained score, but this model predicts how an infinite number of obtained scores would distribute themselves. We use this model to reason about the one obtained score.

The standard deviation of this theoretical distribution is known as the **standard error of measurement (SEM)**. The most common formula for the SEM is

$$SEM = SD\sqrt{1-r}$$

where r signifies the test's reliability and SD denotes the test's standard deviation for the group on which the r was determined. Hence, if $r = .85$ and $SD = 15$, we would calculate the SEM for that test as 5.8, or approximately 6 points.

We can use the SEM to construct a CI around the obtained score. We can then state, with a certain degree of probability, that the person's true score lies within this CI. Note that the CI falls around the obtained score (O in the model), not around the true score (T), because we never know T.

To construct a CI for a test score, we need the test's SD and reliability coefficient (which together yield the SEM, as indicated in the formula above) and a multiplier based on the probability for the

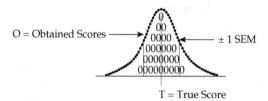

FIGURE 6.2 Hypothetical distribution of many obtained scores (O) around the true score for one individual. SEM = standard error of measurement.

width of the interval. The most common levels of confidence use a multiplier of 1.0, yielding a 68% CI; a multiplier of 1.96, yielding a 95% CI; and a multiplier of 2.58, yielding a 99% CI.

Let us define these CIs for Jonathon, our rambunctious 8-year-old boy with a diagnosis of ADHD. Jonathon's evaluation included an assessment of his intellectual ability with, let us assume, the Wechsler Intelligence Scale for Children, 5th edition (WISC-V). The SD for the WISC-V Fluid Reasoning Index score is 15. Suppose the manual gives the internal consistency reliability for Jonathon's age group as .93. Thus $SEM = 15\sqrt{1-.93}$, or 3.97, which we will round to 4. Jonathon's index score is 110. Let us apply CIs to Jonathon's score:

♦ We have a 68% certainty that Jonathon's true score is 110 ± (1.00 × SEM) = 110 ± 4, or 106–114.
♦ We have a 95% certainty that Jonathon's true score is 110 ± (1.96 × SEM) = 110 ± 8, or 102–118.
♦ We have a 99% certainty that Jonathon's true score is 110 ± (2.58 × SEM) = 110 ± 10, or 100–120.

These represent the most commonly used CIs. You can construct an interval of any width by using different multipliers, which in turn refer to different areas in the normal distribution. A multiplier of 1.65, for example, yields a 90% CI. When referencing the CI for a test score, we will find it important to know whether the interval covers the 68%, 95%, 99%, or perhaps some other percentage interval.

 Skill Exercise 6-1

Suppose a test has $M = 50$, $SD = 10$, and a reliability coefficient $r = .90$. Construct the 95% CI around a score of 40 for this test.

The examples presented for Jonathon's CIs make these handy generalizations clear:

♦ The more confidence you want to have about capturing the true score, the wider the interval you will need to use.
♦ The narrower the interval, the lower your confidence about capturing the true score will be.

♦ The lower the test's reliability, the wider the interval you will want to use.

♦ The higher the reliability, the narrower the interval you will need.

What Reliability Do We Capture With Confidence Intervals?

Talking about *the* reliability of a test will prove misleading. Several sources of unreliability exist, and most reliability coefficients capture only one or a few of those sources. For example, *test–retest reliability* captures unreliability due to temporal fluctuations, but it does not capture unreliability due to differences in test content. *Internal consistency reliability* captures unreliability due to differences in test content, but it does not capture unreliability due to temporal fluctuations. *Generalizability theory* (Brennan, 2001) allows for examining multiple sources of unreliability. However, despite its elegance, generalizability coefficients simply do not exist for most tests. Reliability coefficients capturing only one source of unreliability will prove greater than reliability coefficients covering several sources of unreliability. Since the SEM incorporates the reliability coefficient (see the formula for *SEM*) and the SEM, in turn, enters into the CI, most CIs for test scores presented in test manuals are smaller than they really should be for practical applications. No simple formula exists to correct for this underestimation.

Confidence Intervals for Statistics

We call a descriptive measure (e.g., the mean or a correlation coefficient) on a sample a **statistic**. We call a descriptive measure on an entire population a **parameter**. We use a statistic to estimate a parameter. For example, we use the mean of a sample to estimate the mean of a population; we use a correlation based on a sample to estimate the correlation in the population. The common practice for designating these measures is to represent statistics with ordinary italicized English characters (e.g., *M*, *S*, and *r*) and parameters with Greek letters (e.g., μ [mu], σ [sigma], and ρ [rho]). It is certainly confusing to call a sample's descriptor a "statistic," because we refer to the entire field as "statistics." Nevertheless, statisticians use these as common terminology.

Recognize three facts about this situation. First, we almost always want to know what holds true for a population. For example, we want to know the mean score on the Beck Depression Inventory–II for all postmenopausal women or the correlation between anxiety and depression if we tested everyone in the population. Second, we nearly always have only the information on a sample—in this instance, the sample mean or sample correlation. Third, we use the sample statistic (e.g., *M*) to estimate or draw an inference about the population parameter (e.g., μ).

The **standard error of a statistic** provides an index of the precision with which the statistic estimates its corresponding parameter. Think of many random samples drawn from the population. On each sample, we calculate the statistic of interest. These statistics will form a distribution around the parameter. The distribution may follow the normal curve, as in Figure 6.3.

Let us assume for the moment that the parameter lies at the center of this distribution and that we can determine the distribution's SD. We call the SD of this distribution the *standard error* (SE) *of the statistic*. Note that the SE counts as an SD, but it is not the SD of the original measure (e.g., people's test scores). It is the SD of the means of many samples. With the SE in hand, we can use the properties of the normal curve to make statements about the likelihood that a particular statistic (the one we got for our sample) lies within a certain distance of the parameter. Figure 6.3 shows a distribution of sample means around the population parameter μ.

A CI creates a region around a statistic with the expectation that the parameter corresponding to the statistic falls within that region with a certain degree of probability. Confidence intervals suggest

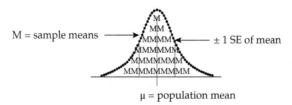

M = sample means → ← ± 1 SE of mean

μ = population mean

FIGURE 6.3 Distribution of sample means (*M*) around the population parameter μ. SE = standard error.

[M   ]   2.58 SE = 99% CI   (14–24)

[M   ]   1.96 SE = 95% CI   (15–23)

   [M]   1.00 SE = 68% CI   (17–21)

+++
2 4 6 8 10 12 14 16 18 20 22 24 26 28 30 32 34 36 38 40

FIGURE 6.4 Illustration of confidence intervals (CIs) for a mean $M = 19$ and a standard error $SE = 2$.

how much "wobble" might occur in using the statistic to estimate a parameter. As was the case for the CI for a test score, as described above, we will often find CIs for statistics given for the 68%, 95%, and 99% levels. Figure 6.4 shows a graphic presentation of CIs for a mean (M) of 19 and SE of 2.

We have illustrated the concept of an SE and its corresponding CI with the sample mean and the population mean. The same concepts apply to any statistic and its corresponding parameter. However, not all statistics yield a normal or even a symmetrical sampling distribution. We must investigate the nature of the sampling distribution for each statistic. Once we have handled this matter, the concepts of SE and CI apply.

 Skill Exercise 6-2

Suppose we have a sample mean $M = 50$, $SD = 10$, and SE of $M = 3$. Construct the 95% CI around $M = 50$.

Effect Size

The results of tests of statistical significance, as outlined in Chapter 5, depend heavily on the size of the samples (N, N_1, N_2, etc.). Given a sufficiently large sample size, almost any difference in means or any degree of correlation will qualify as statistically significant. Beware of such declarations as "significant" and "highly significant" with large or unspecified sample sizes.

Consider a hypothetical example involving the comparison of male and female alcohol abusers (denoted as groups 1 and 2, respectively) with means $M_1 = 50$ and $M_2 = 52$ and with $SD = 10$ for each group. If N_1 and N_2 were each 25, the *t*-test would yield $t = .70$, a clearly nonsignificant difference. However, if N_1 and N_2 were each 1,000, the *t*-test would yield $t = 4.47$, a clearly significant difference, with $p < .001$. We must temper our interpretation of this "highly significant" result by the observation that a 2-point difference on the measure of alcohol abuse may possess little practical importance. This illustrates the oft-cited difference between "statistically significant" and "clinically significant."

We can observe the same kinds of results when working with other hypothesis tests. Large sample sizes may produce statistically significant results that have little practical meaning. For this reason, we want to supplement a hypothesis test with some measure of effect size.

Measures of **effect size (ES)** express the degree of difference between group means or the degree of correlation between variables *independent of the sample size*. Although many journals have policies encouraging use of ES measures, the editors rarely enforce such policies consistently. Furthermore, even when an original article reports measures of ES, they often become lost when the results from the article are summarized elsewhere. Intelligent interpretation of results always requires application of the notion of ES—if not formally, at least informally.

Two Common Measures of Effect Size

There are two frequently used measures of ES, as well as a host of others. The first is *d*, sometimes called **Cohen's *d*,** although variations on Cohen's version exist, with other names attached. The most common variation is Hedge's *g*; even when calculated according to Hedge's formula, sources often refer to the result as *d*. The simplest case of *d* is

$$d = \frac{M_T - M_C}{SD}$$

where M_T and M_C are the means of the treatment and control groups, respectively, and SD represents the pooled SD for the two groups (or, in one version of *d*, simply the SD of the control group). For example, if M_T = 25, M_C = 20, and SD = 10, then d = 0.5. We provide further examples of d below. In the medical literature, as well as in some other contexts, what we have described here as d is often called the **standardized mean difference**, with the acronym SMD.

 Skill Exercise 6-3

This exercise comes in two parts, both related to measures of ES.

Numerous websites now provide calculators for ES. To see some of them, enter "effect size calculator" in any Internet search engine. Open a couple of them to see how they work.

Recall the Campbell Collaboration database of evidence-based reviews described in Chapter 3. Go to its own ES calculator at www.campbellcollaboration.org/resources/effect_size_input.php. Click on "Standardized Mean Difference (d)," then on "Means and standard deviations." Enter these data for Mean, SD, and N: Treatment 52, 10, 40; Control 50, 10, 45. What is d? Does the 95% CI include 0.0? Try some other data for Mean, SD, and N.

The second common measure of ES is simply the correlation coefficient (r), a number confined to the range −1.00 to +1.00, constituting a self-defining measure of ES. For example, an r of .95 is very high; an r of .10 is very low. Many researchers and readers of research simply square the r value (r^2) to obtain an informal ES. For example, an r of.60 yields an r^2 of .36, meaning 36% of the variance is accounted for.

Importantly, the sample size N affects the statistical significance of r. Note that N enters into the formula for determining the SE of r, which in turn enters into the hypothesis test. As above, a large N can yield a "highly significant" r that does not have much practical importance. For example, r = .04 attains significance at the .001 level when based on N = 10,000. But r = .04 will prove worthless for practical purposes. Similarly, r = .15 based on 500 cases rates as significant at the .001 level but is of little practical value.

	Small	Medium	Large
d	.20	.50	.80
r	.10	.30	.50

FIGURE 6.5 Summary of Cohen's benchmarks for *d* and *r* as effect sizes.

Benchmarks for Measures of Effect Size

Cohen (1988) offered a series of **effect size benchmarks** for the interpretation of *d* and *r*. Often researchers refer to these as "Cohen's benchmarks." Although intended as informal guides, these designations have struck a resonant chord in the research community and have won adoption with surprising consensus. Figure 6.5 lists these benchmarks.

Graphic Illustrations of Effect Size

Keeping these benchmarks for measures of ES in mind will prove useful, but you may find it even more useful to draw the measures of ES and keep the drawings in mind when interpreting research results. Figure 6.6 illustrates the three benchmark measures for *d*. As shown there, with *d* = 0.20 there is almost complete overlap between the two distributions, for example, between a treatment and a control group. Even *d* = 0.80 shows quite a bit of overlap. To achieve almost complete separation between the two distributions requires a *d* of

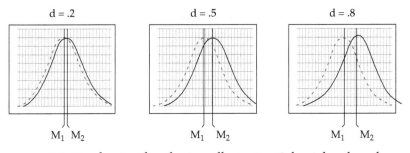

FIGURE 6.6 Overlapping distributions illustrating Cohen's benchmarks for small, medium, and large effect sizes.

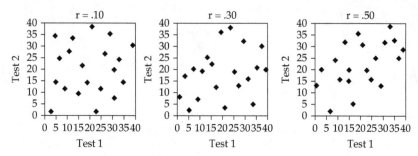

FIGURE 6.7 Scattergrams illustrating Cohen's benchmarks for small, medium, and large effect sizes *r*.

approximately 6, an ES hardly ever found in behavioral health and addiction research. For example, when reading about an "evidence-based" treatment for which the investigator claims much more effectiveness than a control or waiting list, one might expect a *d* of 0.80, a large ES according to the customary benchmarks.

Figure 6.7 shows examples of correlation scattergrams for the three benchmarks for *r*. For *r* = .10, one can barely detect a relationship between the two variables by the naked eye. For *r* = .50, one can clearly detect the drift of points from lower left to upper right, although the relationship hardly qualifies as perfect. Note that the verbal descriptions for these benchmarks for *r* as an ES do not apply to measures of reliability. We have much higher standards for reliability. For example, we would consider a reliability of .50 very low.

 Skill Exercise 6-4

Suppose you have a mean of a treatment group $M_T = 60$ and mean of the control group $M_C = 50$, with both groups having $SD = 10$. Construct overlapping distributions, such as those in Figure 6.6, to illustrate the measure of effect size *d*.

Additional Descriptors of Effect Size

Table 6.1 presents additional ways to interpret measures of ES. The left-hand column shows the traditional measure of effect size *d*, as

TABLE 6.1 Alternative Frameworks for Interpreting Measures
of Effect Size

Effect size (ES or *d*)	Percentile of treated patients	Success rate of treated patients	Type of effect	Cohen's standard
1.00	84	72%	Beneficial	
0.90	82	70%	Beneficial	
0.80	79	69%	Beneficial	Large
0.70	76	66%	Beneficial	
0.60	73	64%	Beneficial	
0.50	69	62%	Beneficial	Medium
0.40	66	60%	Beneficial	
0.30	62	57%	Beneficial	
0.20	58	55%	Beneficial	Small
0.10	54	52%	No Effect	
0.00	50	50%	No Effect	
−0.10	46	<50%	No Effect	
−0.20	42	<50%	Detrimental	
−0.30	38	<50%	Detrimental	

described above, for treated versus untreated or wait-list patients. The second column shows the percentile rank of the average treated patient in comparison with untreated patients for each level of ES. For example, with an ES of 0.60 in favor of a treatment, the average patient in the treatment group would stand at the 73rd percentile in the untreated group. The third column shows the success rate of treated patients in comparison with untreated patients. The fourth column provides a "common sense" descriptive label for the numerical indicators. The right-hand column applies the Cohen benchmarks.

Other Measures of Effect Size

The two most commonly used measures of ES are *d* and *r*, but researchers employ a host of other measures, each one developed to accompany a particular type of statistical analysis. The intent of each of these other measures is the same: to give some sense of the meaningfulness of results apart from tests of statistical significance, which depend excessively on sample size.

Simple formulas allow for conversion between many of the measures of ES. For example, we can convert Cohen's *d*, expressing the difference between two group means, to a *point biserial correlation* (a variation of the usual Pearson correlation where one variable, in this case group membership, has a value of 0 or 1). Such conversions prove helpful when comparing results from different studies. For example, one study may express its results as correlation coefficients, while another study presents *t*-tests. Thus these conversions frequently appear in meta-analyses, which combine results from many studies.

 The book's companion website contains a list of many measures of ES and formulas for converting between them.

Interpreting Results as Proportion of Variance in Common

A popular way to interpret a variety of research results involves focusing on the **proportion of variance in common**. When results appear as correlation coefficients (*r*, *R*), the square of the coefficient (r^2, R^2) tells the proportion of variance in common between the variables, as described above. For example, with $r = .50$ between a measure of anxiety and a measure of depression, we say that the two measures have 25% (i.e., $.50^2$) of their variance in common. We can translate results of *t*-tests, *F*-tests, and χ^2 tests into correlation form to use this same method of interpretation.

It may prove useful to think about this method of interpretation graphically. Figure 6.8 shows how to do this in the case of *r*; it works equally well for *R* (multiple correlation). In the left-hand panel of Figure 6.8, the two variables overlap very substantially, in fact, almost completely. We find little that is unique to either variable. In the middle panel, the two variables overlap by about one-half. In the right-hand panel, not very much exists in common between the two variables, corresponding to a very modest *r* of roughly .30.

Using proportion of variance in common as a method of interpretation often gives rise to conflicting viewpoints on an issue. Consider

90% overlap	50% overlap	10% overlap
$r^2 = .90$	.50	.10
$r = .95$	.71	.32

FIGURE 6.8 Illustration of percent overlap in the variance for two variables.

the case of $r = .30$, which is "medium" according to Cohen's benchmarks for r but corresponds to only 9% variance in common, which sounds almost negligible. Or consider $r = .50$, which seems, on the face of it, a respectable correlation and in fact qualifies as "large" according to Cohen's benchmarks. However, it accounts for only 25% of the variance, leaving 75% of the variance as nonoverlapping between the two variables. Remain cognizant of these interpretive difficulties as you peruse the research literature.

A measure of ES that often accompanies results of an analysis of variance goes by the rather unusual name of η^2 (read as "eta squared"; the letter that looks somewhat like an "n" is actually the Greek letter eta). Like r^2, it gives the proportion of variance accounted for. However, interpreting η^2 can prove a bit tricky when it arises from comparison of three or more groups. A particular η^2 may seem quite robust, but you need to examine the array of means to see what is "really going on." A related measure, partial η^2, results from a design with more than one independent variable (see "Factorial Designs" in Chapter 5). Partial η^2 uses concepts like partial correlation (see Chapter 5) to assign a percentage of variance to an independent variable exclusive of the effects of other independent variables.

Rates, Ratios, Sensitivity, Specificity, and Predictive Power

Behavioral health and addiction research often refers to a host of rates, ratios, and derivative measures. In this section, we identify the most frequently used indexes within this plethora of percentages and provide examples of interpretation for each index.

Prevalence Rates and Related Ratios

A **prevalence rate** identifies the percentage of a population having a particular characteristic. For example, the prevalence rate for autism spectrum disorder approximates 0.5–0.8% in the general population of the United States (Karpiak & Zaboski, 2013). Writers in the clinical literature usually prefer the term *prevalence rate*, but in other contexts, the term **base rate** carries the same meaning.

Separate prevalence rates may apply for persons who (a) have the characteristic at any one time or (b) have ever had the characteristic. We can usually define the former type of prevalence rate for a certain period of time, one common period being 1 year (giving us the *1-year prevalence rate*). Or the period might be "right now." The percentage of the population who have ever had the characteristic constitutes the *lifetime prevalence rate*.

Distinguishing among these various uses of the term becomes crucial. Consider how the percentages (prevalence rates) would change in answer to these questions: Do you currently abuse alcohol? Have you abused alcohol in the past 12 months? Have you ever abused alcohol, even in adolescence or early adulthood?

When examining research literature, keep several important points in mind about prevalence rates:

♦ As just noted, you should distinguish carefully between the one-time and the lifetime definitions of prevalence rate. They can differ substantially, and often do.

♦ Be careful about drawing conclusions about prevalence rates in entire populations when comparing the prevalence rates between two groups. For example, bulimia nervosa may occur 10 times more often in women than in men. That sounds dramatic and has great clinical significance. But it does not mean that most women will likely suffer from that condition. Similarly, boys are 3 times more likely than girls to manifest ADHD. That does not mean the typical boy has ADHD. We expand on this matter of comparing prevalence rates later.

♦ Varying prevalence rates can have a substantial impact on test validity, especially when we use a test for purposes of selection or identification. Suppose we use a test to identify persons likely to attempt suicide. The one-time prevalence rate for this characteristic is quite low, less than 1%. No matter how good the test, we will likely maximize correct classifications (attempters vs. nonattempters) by simply classifying everyone as a nonattempter. That is not helpful in a clinical context. Or consider the case in which a characteristic's prevalence rate is high (e.g., 90% of college students drink alcohol). Using a test to distinguish between students who will or will not use alcohol is virtually hopeless. Simply predict that everyone will drink and you will guess correctly 90% of the time—hard odds to beat. Test validity, in the sense of usefulness of the test for identification, tends to be maximized when prevalence rates reach a moderate level, the best case being 50%.

♦ Prevalence rates can vary substantially among subgroups, a fact that has important implications for the potential effectiveness of tests. For example, while the prevalence rate for suicide attempters runs less than 1%, the prevalence rate for attempters among individuals who score above a certain point on a measure of depression may jump to 30%. Within that group, a test might prove very helpful in identifying attempters in clinical contexts.

Internet searches for "base rate" or "prevalence rate" AND "(name of disorder)" will yield much useful information. The US National Institute of Mental Health (NIMH) provides summaries of prevalence rates for many disorders at www.nimh.nih.gov/health/statistics/prevalence/index.shtml. Other useful websites include those of the US Centers for Disease Control and Prevention (CDC) and the World Health Organization (WHO).

 Skill Exercise 6-5

Enter in any Internet search engine "prevalence AND autism." Check the CDC and WHO websites for prevalence rates and trends. Then do likewise for other mental and addictive disorders of interest.

Odds Ratio and Relative Risk

A variety of techniques assist with comparisons of prevalence rates among groups. We note increasing use of the **odds ratio** (OR),

TABLE 6.2 Hypothetical Data to Illustrate Use
of Odds Ratio

	No. of ADHD cases	No. of non-ADHD cases	Total cases
Boys	16	175	191
Girls	5	190	195
Total cases	21	365	386

shorthand for the more complete term "ratio of conditional odds" (Kennedy, 1992). Let's apply the technique to a comparison of ADHD in boys and girls in a school system (see Table 6.2). We created hypothetical data, and for simplicity, we disregard the subtypes of ADHD.

We express odds as the ratio of number of favorable outcomes to number of unfavorable outcomes. If you roll an unbiased die, the probability that you will get a 6 is 1/6, but the odds of getting a 6 are 1:5 (read "one to five"), assuming 6 is a favorable outcome. In our hypothetical example, the odds that a boy has ADHD are 16:175. The odds that a girl has ADHD are 5:190. These odds can be written as 16/175 for boys and 5/190 for girls. We can then calculate the OR as the ratio for boys divided by the ratio for girls, resulting in OR = 3.47. Put into words, boys are about three and a half times more likely than girls to suffer from ADHD.

When two groups under comparison have the same prevalence rates, OR = 1.00. As the rate in the first group (in the numerator) becomes increasingly greater than the rate in the second group (in the denominator), the OR can become infinitely large. As the rate in the first group becomes increasingly smaller than the rate in the second group, the OR approaches 0.

Switching the positions of the groups (i.e., whether the first or second group is in the denominator) results in the OR's moving above or below its central value of 1. However, the one OR will equal the reciprocal of the other. In our ADHD example, using the ratio for boys as the numerator and the ratio for girls as the denominator yielded OR = 3.47. Reversing numerator and denominator gives OR = 0.288 (i.e., girls have less than a third the likelihood of an ADHD diagnosis as boys). Note that 3.47 and .288 are reciprocals of each other (1/3.47 = 0.288 and 1/0.288 = 3.47).

The OR is asymmetrical around its "equal point" of 1.0. Below 1, the OR can go only to 0, so values in that range do not appear startling. Above 1, OR values can go to infinity, and even values like 15 or 20 do seem startling. Translating ORs back and forth using the reciprocal relationship helps to counteract this disparity in viewpoints.

We usually find a specific OR accompanied by a CI, most commonly a 95% CI. The **OR confidence interval** is determined by log transformation and therefore will not seem obvious to the nonmathematician. However, we interpret the OR confidence interval in the usual way: It provides a range within which the "true OR" probably falls. Since an OR of 1 means equal odds for the two groups, we must ask the crucial question of whether an OR's confidence interval includes 1.00. If it does, then no important difference may exist between the odds for the two groups. And like all CIs, the OR's confidence interval is heavily dependent on the number of cases in the groups involved in calculating the OR. Small numbers of cases result in wide CIs for the OR; large numbers of cases result in narrow CIs.

Relative risk (RR), also known as the *risk ratio*, offers another way to compare prevalence in two groups. Like the OR, RR is a ratio, but a ratio of the actual prevalence rates in the two groups. Consider the data in Table 6.2. The risk of ADHD for boys is 16/191 (number of boys with ADHD divided by total number of boys), or .084. The risk of ADHD for girls is 5/195 (number of girls with ADHD divided by total number of girls), or .026. The *relative* risk of ADHD for boys (in comparison with girls) is .084/.026 = 3.23. The *relative* risk of ADHD for girls (in comparison with boys) is .026/.084. = 0.31. The RR for boys is the reciprocal of the RR for girls.

Four characteristics of RR correspond to characteristics of the OR. First, the "balance point," where the rates are equal in two groups, is 1.0. Second, on the high side both measures can go to infinity, while on the low side they can go only to 0. Third, as for the OR, RR in one direction is the reciprocal of RR in the other direction. Fourth, we can construct a CI for RR. It too relies on logarithms, and once again, the key question is whether the CI includes 1.0.

Still another common-sense way to compare the two groups uses the *risk difference*. This simply equals the raw difference in rates for the two groups. In our example, the risk for boys is .084 and the risk for girls is .026, yielding a risk difference of .058. That is, boys are more at risk for ADHD by a difference of .058.

Skill Exercise 6-6

Cover up the bottom part of this table, looking only at the top part in bold font. Use what you have learned to calculate the OR, RR, and risk difference for ADHD in boys versus girls. Then uncover the bottom part of the table to check yourself.

	ADHD	Non-ADHD	Total
Boys	**20**	**180**	**200**
Girls	**4**	**96**	**100**
Total	**24**	**276**	**300**
Odds ratio	Odds for boys	20/180	0.111
	Odds for girls	4/96	0.042
	OR	(20/180)/(4/96)	2.667
Risk ratio	Risk for boys	20/200	0.100
	Risk for girls	4/100	0.040
	RR	(20/200)/(4/100)	2.500
Risk difference	Risk for boys	20/200	0.100
	Risk for girls	4/100	0.040
	Risk difference	(20/200) − (4/100)	0.060

Sensitivity, Specificity, and Predictive Power

Consider a test designed to identify ADHD patients. More precisely, the test needs to distinguish between ADHD cases and non-ADHD cases. Let's call the ADHD cases the *target group*. Contrasts between any condition and the absence of the condition, for example, depressed and nondepressed or cocaine user and nonuser, would serve equally well for illustrating the following points.

The concepts of sensitivity and specificity describe the efficiency with which the test distinguishes the target group from the nontarget group. **Sensitivity** refers to the percentage of cases correctly identified as falling within the target group. Some sources use the term *selectivity* as an equivalent to sensitivity. **Specificity** refers to the percentage of cases correctly identified as falling within the nontarget group.

Determining sensitivity and specificity requires the use of a **cut score** on the test. We tag people above the cut score as belonging to the target group. We tag people below the cut score as not belonging to the target group. In this instance, high scores on the test indicate presence of ADHD. A test using binary scores (e.g., 1 vs. 0 or Yes vs. No) has a built-in cut score. Most tests used in clinical practice have a continuous scale, but it becomes a binary system (above vs. below) when we apply the cut score.

Figure 6.9 illustrates the application of a cut score to our test designed to identify ADHD patients. It shows the cut score, set here at 16+, applied to distributions of scores for ADHD and non-ADHD cases. We assume that careful evaluation of the patients has resulted in correct placement in their respective groups. This assumption often

Test Score	Group	
	ADHD	Non-ADHD
20	1	
19	2	
18	6	8
17	9	12
16	12	20
15	10	60
14	6	40
13	3	24
12	1	16
11		12
10		8
Total	50	200

Sensitivity = 60% (brace spanning test scores 20–16)

Specificity = 80% (brace spanning test scores 15–10)

FIGURE 6.9. Hypothetical distributions of test scores illustrating sensitivity and specificity.

proves tenuous in actual practice. For example, the non-ADHD group may contain some real ADHD cases that have simply escaped notice. (Refer to Figure 8.1 for a sample decision tree on Jonathon's ADHD diagnosis.) Conversely, the ADHD group may contain some incorrectly diagnosed cases. However, we make the assumption of correct classification to develop the notions of sensitivity and specificity.

In Figure 6.9, the test's sensitivity is 60% (i.e., 60% of the ADHD cases scored above the cut score). The test's specificity is 80% (i.e., 80% of the non-ADHD cases fell below the cut score and we correctly identified them as non-ADHD). Notice that using a cut score of 16+ means that we "missed" 40% of the ADHD cases and incorrectly tagged 20% of the non-ADHD cases as ADHD.

Observe what happens if we move the cut score down to 15+ with the hope of capturing more of the ADHD cases. That move does indeed capture more ADHD cases, improving sensitivity from 60% to 80%. However, we have simultaneously decreased specificity from 80% to 50%. Because there is an inevitable trade-off between sensitivity and specificity, we should always present them together.

Now consider these extreme cases: If we set the cut score at 12+, we have a wonderful-looking sensitivity of 100%, but specificity plunges to 10%—we classify 90% of the non-ADHD cases as ADHD. At the other extreme, setting the cut score at 19+ yields a marvelous specificity of 100%, but sensitivity plummets to 6%—we miss 94% of the ADHD cases.

Let us convert Figure 6.9 to a 2 × 2 table (Table 6.3), classifying cases only as at or above and below the cut score of 16+ for the ADHD and non-ADHD groups. With the information in this format, we can introduce the notions of positive and negative predictive power. **Positive predictive power** (PPP) refers to the percentage of actual ADHD cases out of all the cases falling at or above the cut score. In Table 6.3, this is 30/70 = 43%. **Negative predictive power** (NPP) refers to the percentage of non-ADHD cases out of all cases falling below the cut score. In Table 6.3, this is 160/180 = 89%. Thus based on these data, there is approximately a 40% chance that a previously unevaluated child with a score of 16+ is ADHD. Approximately a 90% chance exists that previously unevaluated child without ADHD with a score of less than 16 is non-ADHD.

Obviously, placement of the cut score affects PPP and NPP, with the effects generally going in opposite directions. The effect of the prevalence rate for the condition is not as obvious. As noted earlier, however, when a condition has an extremely low prevalence rate, identifying cases with the condition becomes difficult indeed. Thus both sensitivity and PPP will typically prove poor.

 Skill Exercise 6-7

Go to the website www.medcalc.org/calc/diagnostic_test. php. Enter the data from Table 6.3. Verify PPP and NPP. Notice the other indicators that the site automatically calculates for you.

False Positives and False Negatives

We often use the terms *false positive* and *false negative* in the clinical literature to describe the relationship between test performance and an external criterion. The external criterion might require a thorough evaluation resulting in a diagnosis, such as whether a person is depressed or nondepressed or is successful or not successful. The relationship between standing on the test and standing on the external criterion may appear as shown in Figure 6.10. The figure shows classification of individuals into depressed and nondepressed cases based on careful evaluation and diagnosis and on their test performance, specifically in terms of whether they scored above or below a cut score. In this example, a high score is indicative of depression.

TABLE 6.3 ADHD and Non-ADHD Cases Above and Below Cut Score for Figure 6.9

	No. of ADHD cases	No. of non-ADHD cases	Total cases	Predictive power
Above cut score	30	40	70	PPP = 30/70 = 43%
Below cut score	20	160	180	NPP = 160/180 = 89%

Note: NPP = negative predictive power; PPP = positive predictive power

Test Performance

	Below	Above
Depressed	False Negative 5	Hit 15
Not Depressed	Hit 65	False Positive 15

Cut-score on Test

FIGURE 6.10 False positives, false negatives, and hits in a 2 × 2 configuration for a hypothetical test.

False positive cases are those that fall above the cut score on the test but in fact do not suffer from depression (i.e., people that the test wrongly categorized as depressed). **False negative** cases are those that fall below the cut score on the test but are truly depressed (i.e., people that the test wrongly categorized as not depressed). **Hits** are cases where the test classification and the external criterion classification agree. Either the test identified them as depressed and they indeed qualify as depressed according to the external criterion, or the test identified them as nondepressed and they indeed qualify as nondepressed. Some sources call the former hits, in the upper right quadrant of Figure 6.10, *true positives*. Correspondingly, we would call the latter hits, in the lower left quadrant, *true negatives*, because the test correctly identified these people as not depressed.

Placement of the cut score clearly affects all the numbers in the figure. Most importantly, increasing the cut score (moving it to the right in Figure 6.9) will decrease the number of false positives but simultaneously increase the number of false negatives. Similarly, as a general rule, decreasing the cut score will decrease the number of false negatives but increase the number of false positives. We can see many similarities between this way of looking at classification decisions and the treatment of sensitivity and specificity described earlier.

Outliers

The term **outlier** signifies an aberrant data point, one that lies well outside other data points in a distribution or in a configuration of data points. A *univariate* outlier is a data point that lies noticeably far out in a single distribution. A *bivariate* outlier is a data point noticeably outside the *pattern* formed by the data points in an array, for example, in a scattergram. A bivariate outlier may fall within the normal range of data points for each of its variables but outside the pattern formed by the two variables together.

Several definitions of a univariate outlier (Hogan & Evalenko, 2006) rely on the SD, defining an outlier as a point 2 or 3 *SDs* beyond the mean. The most common definition of an outlier (Tukey, 1977) uses the *interquartile range*. Although such formal numerical techniques commonly apply, outliers are pretty easy to spot with the naked eye if you examine the data graphically.

These definitions of outliers refer to individual cases in individual research studies. We also encounter outliers for statistics, including measures of ES, when summarizing results from many studies. A meta-analysis of ESs for cognitive–behavioral therapy, for example, might identify an aberrant result—one much higher or lower than the ESs reported in the other studies.

What does all this have to do with EBPs? Outliers can have a pernicious effect on data summaries, particularly when one is dealing with small samples. An outlier can artificially magnify or diminish the results of systematic reviews and meta-analyses.

What should you look for, then, when interpreting research results? Look for evidence that the authors examined the data for outliers. If they did, you can probably safely rely on their judgment as to whether to include the outlying data points in their data analysis or not. If the authors do not address outliers, then keep in mind that outliers lurking in the data might have a profound effect on their conclusions, especially for small samples.

Checklist for Reading Research

The following summarizes this chapter's recommendations for interpreting numbers commonly seen in research:

- ◆ When interpreting test scores for individuals, apply the SEM to create a CI.
- ◆ When interpreting a statistic, such as a mean, apply the SE of the statistic to create a CI.

♦ When interpreting tests of statistical significance (e.g., of the difference between a treatment and a control group), apply the concept of ES to help determine practical significance.

♦ Apply the benchmarks for measures of ES (*d* and *r*) to aid interpretation.

♦ When examining prevalence rates, make sure you know the time frame used for defining the rate (e.g., now, within the past year, or over a lifetime).

♦ Use the OR, RR, or risk difference to aid in interpreting differences in prevalence rates between groups.

♦ Consider sensitivity and specificity, false positives and false negatives, and PPP and NPP to interpret the effectiveness of a test in separating groups. Recognize the effect of the placement of cut scores in creating trade-offs between these contrasting categories.

♦ Be alert to the possible influence of outliers on summaries of data, especially with small samples.

Key Terms

base rate
Cohen's *d*
confidence interval (CI)
cut score
effect size (ES)
effect size benchmarks
error score
false negatives
false positives
hits
negative predictive power
obtained score
odds ratio
OR confidence interval
outlier

parameter
positive predictive power
prevalence rate
proportion of variance
 in common
relative risk
sensitivity
specificity
standard error of a statistic
standard error of
 measurement (*SEM*)
standardized mean difference
statistic
true score

Answers to Selected Skill Exercises

 Skill Exercise 6-1

SEM = 6.2 (round to 6)

$CI_{.95}$ = 34–46

 Skill Exercise 6-2

SEM = 3 × 1.96 = 5.88 (round to 6)

$CI_{.95}$ = 44–56

 Skill Exercise 6-3

d = 0.20

Yes, $CI_{.95}$ includes 0.0.

Recommended Readings and Websites

Cohen, J. (1988). *Statistical power analysis for the behavioral sciences* (2nd ed.). Hillsdale, NJ: Erlbaum.

Cumming, G. (2012). *Understanding the new statistics: Effect sizes, confidence intervals, and meta-analysis.* New York, NY: Routledge.

Grissom, R. J., & Kim, J. J. (2012). *Effect sizes for research: Univariate and multivariate applications* (2nd ed.). New York, NY: Taylor & Francis.

Karpiak, C. P., & Zaboski, B. A. (2013). Lifetime prevalence of mental disorders in the general population. In G. P. Koocher, J. C. Norcross, & B. A. Greene (Eds.), *Psychologists' desk reference* (3rd ed., pp. 3–16). New York, NY: Oxford University Press.

Medcalc [a useful site for calculating NPP, PPP, selectivity, and sensitivity], www.medcalc.org/calc/diagnostic_test.php

National Institute of Mental Health. (2016). What is prevalence? [a useful site for obtaining prevalence rates]. www.nimh.nih.gov/health/statistics/prevalence/index.shtml

Tukey, J. W. (1977). *Exploratory data analysis.* Reading, MA: Addison-Wesley.

7

Appraising Research Reports

T HE TYPICAL PRACTITIONER WILL TAKE, ON AVERAGE, 15–30 minutes to electronically access the research literature as described in Chapters 3 and 4. Depending on the type (filtered vs. unfiltered) and number (one meta-analysis vs. a bunch of original articles) of information sources, the practitioner will devote anywhere from 15 minutes to three hours to reading and digesting that research information. Now, armed with knowledge of research designs and measures (Chapters 5 and 6), the practitioner stands prepared to engage in **critical appraisal**. This process entails assessing and interpreting research evidence by systematically considering its relevance to the individual clinician's work (Parkes et al., 2001).

In this chapter, we concentrate on the first part of this process: assessing and interpreting research reports. We begin with a description of the individual research article and next consider summaries of reports, especially meta-analytic reviews. Then we examine the problems you should consider for all types of research reports, regardless of design or statistical analysis.

Individual Articles

Individual articles appear in professional, peer-reviewed journals but also in technical reports from research institutes. Principal difficulties with the individual research report include the following:

♦ Each report usually represents only one study or a closely related cluster of similar studies. Such small or unitary studies never "prove" a point. Establishing a solid basis for generalizability requires a whole string of studies, preferably involving different investigators and sites.

♦ Individual research reports reflect biases framed by the investigator's expected results, theoretical allegiances, funding sources, tendency to publish only favorable results, and other extrascientific influences. "Best available research" depends upon a scientific consensus from multiple, independent studies.

♦ Many reports do not provide sufficient detail about the participants and the independent variable (e.g., a treatment) to allow for meaningful interpretation, and especially for understanding possible limitations of the study.

♦ Stated conclusions do not always follow from the data.

Because of the preceding points, one should never rely fully on simply reading the abstract. We return to and expand on these points a little later in the chapter.

Summaries: Narrative Reports and Meta-analyses

The scientific literature typically contains numerous studies on any given topic. For example, thousands of studies have examined the effectiveness of various types of psychotherapy (vs. no therapy or pharmacotherapy). The results of these studies yield varying data and conclusions. To the unsophisticated, these differences feel disconcerting, sometimes suggesting irreconcilable confusion. To those accustomed to conducting research, such differences represent a normal part of science, which seldom appears as simple, clean, and uniform as textbooks on research methods might suggest.

Results may differ simply because of random sampling effects. Results may also differ because of variations in the operational definitions of variables. In psychotherapy, we apply different therapies for varying lengths of time; we define outcomes in terms of changes in test scores in some studies and by self-reports of improvement in other studies; patient samples vary by age, diagnosis, and culture; and so on for other types of differences in detail.

Despite the variations from one study to another, we wish to develop general conclusions about the topic. What generalizations apply to the effectiveness of a given psychotherapy?

Narrative Reviews

The traditional method for developing generalizations from many studies on a single topic is the **narrative review** (or *systematic review*). In this method, the reviewer assembles the relevant studies and then identifies common patterns in the results. The reviewer may discount results that are clearly aberrant or that come from flawed designs. The reviewer may assign special import to studies with particularly strong designs or based on large numbers of cases. In the end, the reviewer provides generalizations about the topic, often with qualifications about softer parts of the research base and with suggestions for further research.

Meta-analyses

Meta-analysis is a statistical technique—or more accurately, a family of statistical techniques—that enables researchers to formally combine or summarize results from many studies on a given topic. Meta-analysis takes the actual results from the relevant studies and aggregates them quantitatively. This technique has the same purpose as the narrative/systematic review: to develop generalizations. Furthermore, both approaches begin the same way (i.e., by assembling relevant studies of the topic). The two approaches differ in the formality of the means by which they combine results.

Prior to the 1980s, summaries in the published literature consisted entirely of the narrative variety. Today, meta-analysis constitutes the industry standard for developing generalizations from multiple studies. Hence every graduate student and practitioner needs to understand the fundamentals of meta-analysis in order to harvest the fruits of the research evidence.

Meta-analyses proceed at varying levels of complexity. Let's begin with two simple examples, then suggest how more complicated methods proceed. A meta-analysis ordinarily summarizes measures of effect size (ES) such as Cohen's d or a correlation coefficient r (see "Effect

Study	r	N
1	.75	100
2	.25	25
3	.40	40
4	.55	35
5	.50	200
Average r = .54		

FIGURE 7.1 Sample meta-analysis for r.

Size" in Chapter 6). At the simplest level, a meta-analysis averages the d or r values, weighted by their respective sample sizes N.

Figure 7.1 shows an example for the correlation coefficient r. Recall the point made earlier that the key problem with the individual journal article arises from its status as just one study. The person who encountered Study 1 in Figure 7.1 would conclude that a strong correlation exists. The person who encountered Study 2 would conclude that only a slight correlation exists. The person who came across both Studies 1 and 2 would feel left in a quandary. The person who looked at the meta-analysis would conclude that r approximates .54, with fluctuations around this value likely due to sampling error or minor differences in study design.

Figure 7.2 shows an example for d. A person who came upon Study 2 first would conclude that the independent variable (treatment) had a rather potent effect. A person who came upon Study 3 would conclude that the same treatment had no effect or perhaps even a slightly deleterious effect. A person who came upon the

Study	d	N
1	.10	100
2	.65	50
3	−.05	50
4	.02	30
5	.35	100
Average d = .23		

FIGURE 7.2 Sample meta-analysis for d.

meta-analysis would conclude that on average, across several studies, the independent variable had a modestly positive impact.

Advanced Meta-analytic Techniques

The simple methods presented above represent bare-bones meta-analyses. More advanced methods include "psychometric meta-analysis" (Hunter & Schmidt, 2015). We hint here at how these work.

Recall from elementary statistics that group heterogeneity affects the magnitude of r (that is, the greater the variability in the group, the higher the value of r, while lesser variability tends to reduce r). We sometimes call this phenomenon the **range restriction** problem. Some relatively simple formulas allow for correcting a given r for differences in group heterogeneity or range. Recall also that reliability restricts validity. Again, some relatively simple formulas, often called **corrections for attenuation**, allow us to correct a given r for imperfect reliability in either or both of the variables involved in a correlation. We might apply either or both types of correction to the data in Figure 7.1 to provide a more sophisticated analysis.

Still another extension of bare-bones meta-analysis, described in more detail below, involves coding characteristics of the studies themselves and then determining whether those characteristics relate systematically to the measures of ES in the studies (r or d). Examples of study characteristics include year of publication, age of patients, and type of dependent variable. Several meta-analyses on the effect of psychotherapy for depression found that investigator allegiance (commitment of the investigator to the type of therapy applied) was associated with the reported effectiveness of the therapy (Prochaska & Norcross, 2014).

We conclude this brief exposition with a few notes on procedural matters. The meta-analytic process starts by assembling the studies for analysis. The typical meta-analysis report describes this process in considerable detail, including a list of the studies. However, the meta-analyst must limit the studies to ones that include the required statistics or, in some instances, that enable the analyst to compute the required statistics from other information in the study. For example, we might convert a d to an r or vice versa using formulas covered in the section on ES in Chapter 6. The entire process may sound quite mechanical. It is not. The analyst must make judgments about which studies qualify for inclusion. Inclusion should not be limited to studies that show significant results; in fact, the significance of results in individual studies should not get them special attention. See the checklist later in this chapter for potential biases in meta-analytic reports.

A report of a meta-analysis often includes a confidence interval (CI) for the average measure of ES. Most reports use a 95% CI. We can interpret such CIs in the same way as CIs for any type of statistic: as a range within which the "true" population value for the measure of ES lies with a certain degree of probability (see Chapter 6 for a full description of CIs).

Typical Methods of Reporting Results of a Meta-analysis

Some reports of a meta-analysis may simply state, "A recent meta-analysis of treatment X showed an average effect size of 0.43." Lurking behind such statements we find a considerable array of tables, graphs, and subanalyses. We highlight here some typical ways of conveying the information from a meta-analysis.

The Forest Plot

Results of a meta-analysis are often displayed graphically in the form of a *forest plot*. Figure 7.3 presents an example of a forest plot based on the data from a simple meta-analysis shown in Table 7.1. The left-hand column (the Y-axis) typically lists the separate studies included in the meta-analysis, most often with author identification, sometimes just serially numbered (1, 2, 3, . . .), as we have done in Figure 7.3. Columns may or may not appear between the list of studies on the left and the actual plot on the right. When columns do appear, they virtually always give the ES and CI (lower and upper limits) for each study—the same information shown visually in the plot. Intermediate columns may also include standard errors, variances, weights, and other statistics derived in the meta-analysis.

The plot shows the ES for each study, with "tails" around the ES showing limits of the CI, and, at the bottom, the average ES, with its CI, for all studies combined. Typically, a small geometric figure (e.g., a square or circle) represents the ES for each study. In some forest

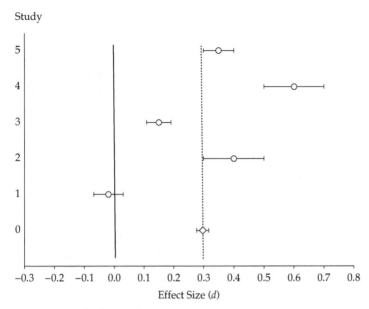

FIGURE 7.3 Sample forest plot.

plots, the size of this figure is proportional to the weight given to the study; other forest plots do not use such scaling by weight.

The X-axis at the bottom of a forest plot varies in two ways. First, it depends on the nature of the ES. It may scale as a Cohen-type *d* or Hedge's *g*, as an odds ratio (*OR*) or risk ratio (*RR*), as a correlation coefficient, or as any other measure of ES. In some instances, it may

TABLE 7.1 Hypothetical Data Used for Constructing the Forest Plot in Figure 7.3

Study	*d*	*SE(d)* × 1.96	LL	*d*	UL
1 Hogan (2010)	−0.02	0.05	−0.070	−0.020	0.030
2 Koocher (2015)	0.40	0.10	0.300	0.400	0.500
3 Maggio (2016)	0.15	0.04	0.110	0.150	0.190
4 Monahan (2016)	0.60	0.10	0.500	0.600	0.700
5 Norcross (2008)	0.35	0.05	0.300	0.350	0.400
Total	0.30	0.02	0.277	0.297	0.317

Note: Studies in first column are sham references. *SE* = standard error; *LL* = lower limit of 95% confidence interval for *d*; *UL* = upper limit of 95% confidence interval for *d*.

show simple percentage. Second, it may be centered on a null ES (e.g., $d = 0.0$ or $OR = 1.0$), or it may be centered on the average ES as determined in the meta-analysis. Sometimes portions of the X-axis are labeled to facilitate interpretation. For example, the words "favors treatment" may appear below the scale for positive values of d and "disfavors treatment" below negative values of d. However, not all forest plots use such verbal labels.

 Skill Exercise 7-1

To see the considerable variety in appearance of forest plots, type "images of forest plots" into any Internet search engine. Click on a few of the forest plots and compare their features. What is plotted (on the X-axis)? What data (if any) accompany the plot?

Indexes of Heterogeneity

In an ideal world, the various studies entering a meta-analysis would show reasonable consistency: The results surely would not be identical, but they would be in the same ballpark. But what really happens? Results may or may not show great consistency. Suppose we are using Hedge's g as our measure of ES, and five studies yield g values of 0.45, 0.50, 0.43, 0.52, and 0.47. That's pretty good consistency. It comports entirely with notions of random sampling differences. Suppose, in contrast, our studies yield g values of 0.45, 1.64, −0.20, 0.10, and 0.99. That would be unsettling, especially if all the studies had respectable sample sizes.

In the world of meta-analysis, we call lack of consistency *heterogeneity*. Some measure of heterogeneity (lack of consistency) will often accompany the meta-analysis report of results. There are three widely used indexes of heterogeneity: Q, I, and τ (tau). I and τ are usually reported in squared form, I^2 and τ^2. Each of the three indexes measures a somewhat different aspect of heterogeneity.

What might excessive heterogeneity, as in our second set of g values, suggest? Perhaps some difference between the studies exists other than random sampling. Perhaps some studies treated one age group, some another age group. Perhaps some involved short-term treatments, others long-term. The large degree of heterogeneity suggests we should look further—which brings us to our next topic.

Moderator Analyses and Meta-regression

Provided we have a sufficient number of studies in the meta-analysis (certainly more than in the simple example presented in Figure 7.3 and Table 7.1), and especially when the degree of heterogeneity raises questions, we wish to examine matters in more detail. There are two current methods for doing so. Both methods require that we have auxiliary information about the studies in the meta-analysis, that is, information other than ESs, CIs for the ESs, and weights. Such other information might include characteristics of the participants (age, gender, diagnosis, etc.) and circumstances of the studies themselves (year of publication, types of outcome measures, experience of therapists, etc.). This information gets coded into the data for the meta-analysis.

We essentially conduct mini-meta-analyses on different subgroups, for example, men versus women, to see if similar results obtain. The basic notion here is analogous to that of interactions in analysis of variance. Does an interaction exist between ES and gender? In the context of meta-analysis, characteristics of the studies may serve as moderators, hence the term *moderator analyses*.

When the auxiliary information consists of a continuous variable, for example, year of publication, we can apply regression techniques. That is, we can use the measure of ES as a dependent variable to be predicted by the auxiliary information. Is there a correlation between magnitude of ES and year of publication? In fact, with several pieces of auxiliary information, we can apply the entire arsenal of partial correlation and multiple correlation techniques—hence the tem *meta-regression*.

The Funnel Plot

In addition to forest plots, a second type of plot sometimes accompanies a meta-analysis. This second type, called a *funnel plot*, has not attracted the same wide adoption as the forest plot. The funnel plot shows the relationship between the measure of ES, placed on the X-axis, and the variance in the measure of ES or, in some cases, simply the sample size N (the primary driver of variance).

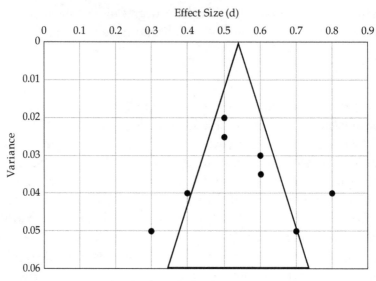

FIGURE 7.4 An example of a funnel plot for studies in a meta-analysis.

Figure 7.4 shows an example of a funnel plot. An odd feature of the funnel plot is that the zero point of the Y-axis sits at the top of the axis rather than its usual position at the bottom of the axis. This arrangement usually results in an upside-down funnel appearance. The funnel plot typically demonstrates that the ESs for studies with the least variance (which ordinarily means the largest numbers of cases) center around the average ES for the meta-analysis, corresponding to the apex of the funnel. Conversely, ESs for studies with larger variances (usually smaller sample sizes) scatter farther from the center. Notice how these tendencies show up in Figure 7.4: The more central ES values, with smaller variances, appear in the "neck" of the funnel, while points with greater variances tend to spread out more around the "top" of the funnel. From a practical perspective, the funnel plot is not nearly as informative as the forest plot.

Publication Bias

A meta-analysis summarizes published studies. "Published" gets broadly defined to include such sources as journal articles, technical reports, and dissertations. But the studies (and their actual statistics) must be publicly available and accessible to the meta-analyst. Despite the rosy picture of the scientific enterprise presented in research methods textbooks, researchers increasingly recognize biases in what gets published. The evidence for such **publication bias** is now overwhelming (van Assen et al., 2015).

One source of publication bias is what we might call the *significance effect*. Authors submit articles only when they get significant results. Reviewers and editors want to publish significant results, not nonsignificant results. Yet, the failure rate for study replication attempts is notoriously high (Anderson & Maxwell, 2016). The cumulative effect of these forces is that meta-analysis summaries may overstate the real-world potency of treatments.

The significance effect is not the only kind of publication bias. Passing fads, political correctness, and assorted other influences impact what gets published. For example, the appearance of a book may make certain kinds of studies more or less publishable (Coburn & Vevea, 2015).

Researchers are developing and applying a host of methods to detect (and possibly correct for) publication bias. Some of the methods involve use of the funnel plot, described above. However, we are a long way from consensus on which methods are best, much less routine application of those methods. Practitioners should be watchful for the possibility of publication bias in meta-analyses. Carefully searching the available literature does not solve the problem. The only studies you can identify are ones that were already published and therefore subject to publication bias.

The Mechanics: Software for Meta-analysis

We'll give just a brief word and some references on the mechanics of "doing the stats" and getting forest plots for meta-analysis. As you might surmise, there are software packages to do the work. First, the Cochrane Collaboration (see Chapter 4) has its own software, called RevMan, which Cochrane reviewers must use but may be used by anyone (tech.cochrane.org/revman/download). Second, Comprehensive Meta-Analysis (www.Meta-Analysis.com) has become a widely used, and widely advertised, commercial software package. Third, most of the major commercial statistical software packages (e.g., SAS, Stata, SPSS) have modules for conducting meta-analysis; in some instances, the module must be purchased separately rather than being part of the standard package. Fourth, R, the free software system, offers add-on packages for conducting meta-analysis.

 Skill Exercise 7-2

Michael Borenstein, chief architect of the Comprehensive Meta-Analysis software just referenced, has some excellent YouTube video explanations of the software. Try this one first—it's about 10 minutes: www.meta-analysis.com/pages/video_overview.php. Then for a longer introduction (60 minutes), try www.youtube.com/watch?v=xWiXeKR3dB4.

Checklist of Potential Methodological Problems with Meta-analytic Reports

The following checklist highlights some possible sources of bias you should be aware of when appraising meta-analyses:

♦ There is potential for bias in the process of locating and selecting studies for inclusion in the analysis.
♦ Studies with significant results are more likely to get published than studies without significant results, leading to publication bias.
♦ Among published studies, those with significant results will more likely win citation by others, and thus become more likely to appear repeatedly.
♦ Bias may be present in sensitivity analyses (analyses of study features potentially related to outcomes, e.g., sample size).

Critical Appraisal of Research Studies

Regardless of the study design, we need to pay attention to the actual conduct of the study to safely draw practice conclusions from it. Furthermore, what we know about the conduct of the study depends on the reporting of the details. For many practical purposes, then, the manner of conducting and reporting the study merges into a single consideration. These concerns apply even to the true experimental design. Five important features of the conduct and reporting of *all* studies require attention: the sample, the independent variable, the dependent variable, the comparison groups, and the relation of the authors' conclusions to the actual results.

The Sample

We need to carefully examine the nature of the patients or cases used in the study. As we have already noted, rarely will a study use a random sample from a meaningful and well-defined population. Even when a randomized clinical trial (RCT) employs random assignment to conditions, the groups in the study rarely originate as random samples from a population. Rather, they typically consist of ad hoc **convenience samples**: We use whomever we can easily recruit.

The practical situation calls for us to turn the textbook problem of inferential statistics upside down. The textbook problem involves having a random sample from a well-defined population and trying to draw an inference from the sample to the population. The practical situation, applicable to nearly all studies in behavioral health and addiction, involves our starting with a convenience sample and having to figure out to what population we can generalize the results.

Estimating to what population we can generalize the results depends critically on having sufficient information about characteristics of the sample. Unfortunately, many reports provide insufficient information in this regard. Prototypically, reports say that the participants studied were "42 depressed students from a Midwestern university" or "76 alcoholabusing clients at a private clinic" without further specification. It proves very difficult—essentially impossible—to generalize from such descriptions to any larger groups.

What information do we want to know? The answer depends on the problem under study. In most circumstances, we would want to know age, gender, racial/ethnic group, socioeconomic status, educational level, and, in treatment studies, mental disorders, previous therapies, readiness for change or motivation, and the like. If specific exclusion criteria applied in the selection of individuals, the report should specify those criteria and describe the effects of applying them (e.g., percentages excluded). The National Institute of Mental Health's Treatment of Adolescent Depression Study (TADS), for example, screened out 85% of the target group of depressed adolescents while still claiming applicability of the results to the entire target group (Westen, 2006).

In some circumstances, information about physical condition, medical status, job classification, family situation, and personal history might be important. For example, if the 42 depressed students at a Midwestern university had all participated in a project on the effects of psychotherapy on their depression, we would certainly want to know about their depression, comorbid diagnoses, current medications, and other important characteristics. In contrast, if the student participants were recruited through a project about the effects of aerobic training, we would want to know about their ages and physical condition.

The **simple random sample** serves as the "benchmark" type of probability sample, but it constitutes only one type. Other probability samples include *stratified samples* and *cluster samples*, and each of these categories has several subcategories. For a given sample size (N), a stratified sample yields a smaller standard error than does simple random sampling to the extent that the basis for stratification relates to the characteristic under study, thus making the strata different on the characteristic. If the basis for stratification does not clearly relate to the characteristic under study, stratified sampling offers no advantage over simple random sampling. For a given N, cluster sampling yields a larger standard error than does simple random sampling to the extent that clusters are internally homogeneous in comparison with the entire population for the characteristic under study. One often encounters studies that apply formulas for the standard error based on simple random sampling when the investigator actually used some other type of sampling (see, e.g., Alf & Lohr, 2007). Still, the most important problem with respect to sampling in behavioral health and addiction research is the use of convenience samples with limited generalizability in the great majority of studies.

For RCTs, questions about the nature of the sample expand to such matters as loss of cases, for a host of reasons, anywhere in the research process. A review of 669 studies representing 83,834 psychotherapy clients determined that 1 in 5 dropped out or prematurely terminated psychotherapy (Swift & Greenberg, 2012). Meta-analyses now routinely describe dropout rates and cases lost to follow-up, obviously an important consideration for any treatment.

To help account for such losses, an increasing number of investigators use the CONSORT (Consolidated Standards of Reporting Trials) flow chart (see Figure 7.5). It begins with "assessed for eligibility ($n =$)" (e.g., 300 women self-referred for chronic depression at a clinic, like Annique). The flow chart then tracks cases through the research process, right up to the point of final data analysis. How well do the final data represent what you started with in the first box? Even research reports that do not formally use such a flow chart still need to address this question. (Also see Table 8.1 for the 25 CONSORT guidelines for RCTs.)

A potential corrective to reporting meta-analytic results for only those participants who have completed treatment (presumably the

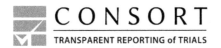

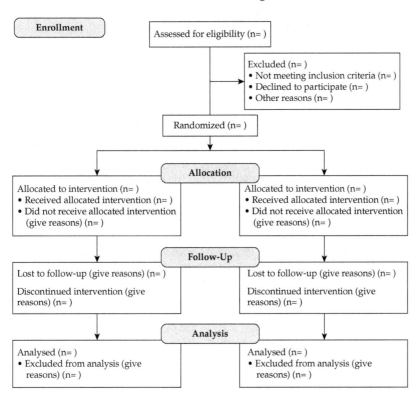

FIGURE 7.5 CONSORT (From Schulz, Altman, Moher, & CONSORT Group, 2010). Distributed under the terms of the Creative Commons Attribution CC BY 2.0.

patients who experienced the most success) involves conducting and reporting an *intent-to-treat* analysis, often referred to as an ITT analysis. This is not so much a single statistical analysis like, say, a *t*-test, but rather a variety of analyses. The general concept goes like this: Consider the bottom row in the Consort flow diagram. That's where you analyze the data from a study. But you started with the second row, where people were randomly assigned to conditions (e.g., treatment or no treatment)—the people you intended to treat, hence the name of the analysis. Do you have the same people in the last analysis row as you had in the allocation row? If not, why not? Did some people not receive the full treatment? Did some people simply disappear? What analyses might you conduct to determine the influence of these changes?

The general problem goes further, although in ways usually not discussed under ITT analysis. You really started in the first row of the diagram with a population. Then some people were deliberately excluded, and others declined to participate. But they were all part of the original group (population) of interest. All these factors need reflection as you look at the final analyses in the last row or in a final report.

The Independent Variable

A huge problem in critically appraising research is *fuzzy definition of the independent variable*. Every study certainly has an independent variable as its focus. For example, a study may compare efficacy of cognitive therapy with a control condition (e.g., no therapy). But if the investigator detects some effect, we always need to ask what really happened. Did the particular cognitive therapy produce the change? Or did the therapeutic relationship, quite apart from the type of therapy, evoke the change? Or did the fact that any therapy took place, regardless of its type, make the difference? Or did the fact that something, almost anything, happened to the people in the treatment group? Authors of a meta-analysis of 32 randomized trials of psychotherapies noted the difficulty of drawing conclusions because "so many of the studies failed to provide necessary information: for example, on therapists . . . , on the interventions . . . and on the location(s)" (Weisz et al., 2006, p. 686).

Customarily, the research literature refers to *the* independent variable as if it constituted a pure, simple element. In behavioral health research, that situation rarely exists. Rather, the independent variable typically includes a complex mixture of elements, much like a chemical compound. For example, a treatment consists of who applies it, under what circumstances, for what length of time, with what degree of fidelity, and so on. Even each of these elements of the independent variable consists of more refined elements. For example, "who" includes the therapist's gender, ethnicity, theoretical orientation, professional discipline, level of training, and interpersonal skills.

Disentangling these elements is no mean feat. Within a single study, it ordinarily proves impossible to isolate all elements of the compound, as we might have the ability to do in the chemistry lab. Nevertheless, when referring to *the* independent variable, we must always remember that it constitutes a complex compound. Thinking in this way allows us to introduce two useful terms, which can be confused because of their phonetic similarity: *mediator* and *moderator*.

Chapter 5 introduced the concept of a mediator (and mediation analysis). Recall that a **mediator** is a variable or factor that makes up the specific mechanism by which a given result happens. It is the causal agent. We now apply that concept in the present context. In our treatment example, the real mediator may be the "who" (the therapist), with all other elements in the compound acting relatively weakly, or it may be the particular therapy method. The mediator may also be the conjunctive force of two of the elements (e.g., length of treatment and therapy method), with either one by itself proving ineffectual and all others proving inert or unimportant. The mediator may also be a spin-off from the treatment situation, such as family members' reactions to the fact that the patient has received treatment.

We distinguish a mediator from a moderator. A **moderator** variable differentiates (in a noncausal sense) the influence of an independent variable. We encountered the notion of moderator earlier in the context of meta-analysis. For example, chronological age may constitute a moderator for the effectiveness of a treatment. For another example, a treatment may be quite effective with recreational cocaine users, somewhat effective for cocaine abusers, and ineffective for chronic cocaine abusers. Detection of moderators becomes one of the principal targets of factorial designs (see Chapter 5) when one of the independent variables is a patient variable.

The Dependent Variable

A third feature of all studies to be critically appraised is the *dependent variable*. It may be off target or less than satisfactory. A treatment may have an effect but not on whatever was operationally defined as the dependent variable; for example, a patient's score on a depression test may have missed the effect. Sometimes the test may prove roughly on target but have such low reliability that the "real effect" becomes swamped by measurement error. Or perhaps the treatment has an effect on the dependent variable, but we have no real interest in that particular dependent variable. For example, the dependent or outcome variable in a study of the effectiveness of psychotherapy will often involve a client's report of satisfaction, but the client's condition may not have actually improved even when he or she says it has (Norcross & Lambert, 2006). We can take pleasure in the fact that the client feels satisfied (one dependent variable), but we would hope that the disorder has diminished (a different dependent variable).

Research reports ordinarily refer to the reliability and validity of the measures used for dependent variables. Treatment of these topics requires special attention. Every clinician or researcher in the behavioral sciences has become familiar with the concepts of reliability and validity for psychological tests. At a general level, *reliability* deals with the consistency of scores, and *validity* deals with what the test actually measures. To interpret research intelligently, we must use greater precision about these terms than what we normally require for a general understanding of them.

Suppose you treat Francesco, the 30-year-old man suffering from generalized anxiety disorder (GAD) and alcohol dependence. You search the literature for treatments for his disorder. The "Method" section of a relevant article says, "GAD was measured with the Scranton Behavior Rating Scale (SBRS), which has demonstrated adequate reliability and validity (Hogan, 2008 [a sham reference here])." Journal policies say that authors should address the reliability and validity of any measures used in the study. The foregoing sentence seems to satisfy that requirement: It gives a citation for the reliability and validity of the test. But does it? The citation refers to the manual for the SBRS, which Hogan authored. Naturally, the manual for the SBRS will report it as a reliable and valid instrument. But what exactly does the manual say?

Readers should remain wary of any blanket statements that a given test is (simply) reliable and valid. No instrument has perfect reliability and validity. Some test authors claim reliability based on rather thin evidence and express satisfaction with reliability levels that would make most people blush. The SBRS may have internal consistency reliability of, say, .75, which makes Hogan quite happy but qualifies as rather marginal in acceptability. Furthermore, the internal consistency reliability of .75 does not tell us anything about the temporal stability of the scores. We must establish the validity of a test for the use of particular scores for particular purposes. What particular scores and what particular purposes were at the root of the test manual's claim of validity?

Although the tests used in a research study are not ordinarily a major focus of attention, the entire array of analyses and conclusions depends critically on their reliability and validity. Low reliability contributes to error variance not only for individual scores but also for group summary statistics. Low reliability leads to low power in the same way that a low number of cases does. Less-than-satisfactory validity means, in essence, that the dependent variable was measured only partially or inappropriately. Thus to make sense of research reports, we need to pay careful attention to the evidence presented for the reliability and validity of the tests used.

The Comparison Group

Textbook descriptions of the RCT design typically present a comparison between a treatment group and a control group. Usually, the treatment receives considerable attention, but the control group merits little comment other than the fact that it is not the treatment. However, from a practical perspective, the nature of the control group is crucial. It deserves careful description by researchers and careful scrutiny by research consumers.

Think of the nature of the control group as falling into one of several categories arranged in a hierarchy of clinical realism (Wampold & Imel, 2015). At the lowest level, the control group gets literally nothing at all. At one step up, the control group has some contact with the researcher. At yet another level up, members of the control group receive a placebo. By **placebo** we mean some action or substance not expected (by the researcher) to exert any real effect. The classic example of a placebo in pharmaceutical studies entails the use of an inert ingredient or a "sugar pill." Thus members of the control group get a pill that looks like the genuine drug but should not have a therapeutic effect.

In the best-designed studies, neither the subjects nor the researchers know who gets the "real" pill (i.e., the supposedly active ingredient) and who receives the placebo. We call this a *double-blind* design. While easily implemented with pills, a double-blind design is challenging to implement in psychotherapy. We can distinguish between a *sham* placebo—a token action of some sort—and a realistic placebo that mimics certain features of the treatment, such as duration and amount of contact.

Another important type of control condition involves **treatment as usual (TAU)**. Here, we contrast the treatment under investigation—the one whose value we seek to establish—with treatment that cases would ordinarily receive in the community. Treatment as usual provides a more realistic contrast than no treatment. We might demonstrate that a new treatment works better than nothing at all, but the real question to ask is whether the new treatment produces better outcomes than what patients would ordinarily exhibit. A research report should describe exactly what TAU entails.

At still higher levels in our hierarchy of control conditions are treatments of structural equivalence (in duration, intensity, amount of contact, etc.) to the treatment under study and, even better, structural equivalence accompanied by researcher allegiance. The latter type of control provides the most rigorous contrast in the investigation of a treatment.

As you read research about the contrast between a treatment and a control group, try to place the control group in the hierarchy just described. The control condition should provide a meaningful contrast with the treatment under investigation. Virtually any treatment can outperform no treatment. The more realistic question is, which of several alternative, structurally equivalent treatments will prove most effective?

Authors' Conclusions Versus Actual Results

The fifth issue to critically consider in appraising all research studies is whether the conclusions the authors draw in the report faithfully follow from the results presented. Making a judgment here requires careful examination of the results related to the conclusions. We often find at least a partial mismatch between data and conclusions— sometimes even a complete mismatch. Researchers, after all, have a vested interest in confirming their research hypotheses. Thus one finds "tendencies, although not significant" or "qualitative observations" turning into firm conclusions. You must also stay alert to hints of causal connections being drawn from designs that do not permit such conclusions.

Consequences of Methodological Malpractice: A Tongue-in-Cheek Lesson

In many research reports, the five concerns outlined above prove more consequential than all the statistical matters that occupy our attention. Let's consider psychotherapy, the most frequent professional activity of behavioral health and addiction professionals. We shall now demonstrate, with tongue firmly planted in cheek, how the preceding concerns can generate spurious conclusions in psychotherapy research studies and outlandish claims in meta-analytic studies about both outcomes (what works) and comparisons among forms of psychotherapy (what works better).

Here are eight ways to inflate your psychotherapy outcome results (success rates or the effect size *d* in meta-analyses) and claim victory for your favored treatment (see Lambert, 2013; Norcross, 2011; Wampold & Imel, 2015, for specifics):

- ◆ *Use only reactive self-report outcome measures.* These tend to change more rapidly (and thus produce bigger gains) than objective measures of life quality, functional status, skill development, and enduring personality change. Assess effectiveness strictly on the basis of clients' short-term satisfaction.
- ◆ *Select highly motivated patients without comorbid conditions.* Require five hours of assessment to weed out the reluctant, begin with the action stage of change to avoid treating those in contemplation, and for goodness' sake, exclude patients with more complex, co-occurring disorders.
- ◆ *Adopt outcome/dependent measures that directly privilege your therapy.* If conducting exposure therapy, for example, use as your

primary measure a behavioral avoidance test responsive specifically to your approach while ignoring other vital measures that perform equally well for multiple therapies. Insist that your therapy works better than others based on the larger ES on your one idiosyncratic measure.

♦ *Compare your favored treatment/independent variable with nothing at all or at least nothing of demonstrated efficacy.* Use a pre–post therapy design to obtain the largest ESs, or if you must, compare your treatment with no treatment or TAU, which frequently equates to no meaningful treatment at all. Then conclude that your treatment produces huge gains for clients and should become the evidence-based therapy of choice.

♦ *Train committed, skilled therapists in your treatment, but don't be so meticulous about any comparison treatments.* In your heart, you already know the alternative treatments are inferior, so just recruit a few graduate students to offer a therapy to which they are neither committed nor skilled. In the final publication, forget to report therapists' commitment to and competence in the alternative treatment.

♦ *Report the outcomes of only those patients completing your treatment.* Avoid the CONSORT transparency requirements (Figure 7.5) and do not chronicle anything on those patients who were excluded from the study, discontinued prematurely, or experienced harm. Only those finishing the study count in the success rates.

♦ *Attribute the success rates entirely to the favored treatment method, not to the therapeutic relationship and certainly not to the patients themselves.* You created the study and you defined the independent variable, so stick to your story: The treatment method alone accounted for the observed improvements!

♦ *Capitalize on extrascientific sources to enhance the success of your treatment.* Follow the evidence in designing, implementing, and publishing your outcome research: Favor your treatment over others (allegiance effect), perhaps even create it yourself (progenitor effect), fund the study through an agency or pharmaceutical company with a vested interest in its success (funding source bias), and publish only when you secure favorable results (publication bias).

Checklist for Appraising Research

Appraising the morass of narrative reviews and meta-analyses requires skills, experience, and a certain level of scrutiny. We hope that you have learned several of these skills and that certain level of scrutiny in this chapter, perhaps especially through the sarcastic counterexamples above. As a reminder about the five important study features to attend to, we provide the following handy checklist.

THE SAMPLE

◆ Does the report adequately describe the sample?
◆ Does the study use a random sample from a clearly defined population?
◆ If the study used a convenience sample, to what population might the results generalize?
◆ Might results of the study prove different for other populations?

THE INDEPENDENT VARIABLE

◆ Does the report adequately describe the independent variable (e.g., a treatment)?
◆ Does the report present evidence or a discussion about which features of the independent variable (e.g., treatment components, therapeutic relationship, homework assignments) might prove crucial?
◆ Do the analyses focus on the independent variable (e.g., a treatment) separately from the person who provided it?

THE DEPENDENT VARIABLE

◆ Does the report adequately describe the dependent variable?
◆ What evidence does the investigator present about the reliability and validity of the measures for the dependent variable?
◆ What effect might unreliability of the dependent variable have on the power of the statistical analysis?
◆ Would alternative definitions of the dependent variable yield similar results?
◆ Did the investigator neglect different dependent variables of possible importance?

THE COMPARISON GROUP

◆ Does the report adequately describe the control condition (comparison group)?
◆ Does the comparison condition make meaningful clinical sense? For example, is it comparable in terms of such factors as length of exposure and therapist allegiance?

RELATION OF CONCLUSIONS TO DATA

◆ Do the data clearly support the conclusions drawn?
◆ Does the investigator make any attempt to draw causal conclusions from a design other than a true experimental design?
◆ Does the report properly qualify groups to which the results might generalize?

This chapter has helped you to understand typical research reports, know how to read them, and determine their value. This wraps up our treatment of the third of the six core steps of EBP, symbolized by the abbreviation AAA TIE (see Chapter 1):

1. Asking a specific, clinical question (Chapter 2)
2. Accessing the best available research (Chapters 3 and 4)
3. Appraising that research evidence critically (Chapters 5–7)
4. Translating that research into practice with a particular patient (Chapter 8)
5. Integrating the clinician's expertise and patient's characteristics, culture, and preferences with the research (Chapter 9)
6. Evaluating the effectiveness of the entire process (Chapter 10).

The fourth step of the EBP process considers the relevance of research evidence to a particular case and applying that evidence in your practice. We turn to that step in Chapter 8.

Key Terms

convenience samples
correction for attenuation
critical appraisal
mediator
meta-analysis
moderator

narrative review
placebo
publication bias
range restriction
simple random sample
treatment as usual (TAU)

Recommended Readings and Websites

Borenstein, M., Hedges, L. V., Higgins, J. P. T., & Rothstein, H. R. (2009). *Introduction to meta-analysis.* Hoboken, NJ: Wiley.

CONSORT 2010 guidelines, www.consort-statement.org/consort-2010

Cumming, G. (2012). *Understanding the new statistics: Effect sizes, confidence intervals, and meta-analysis.* New York, NY: Routledge.

Garson, G. D. (2013). *Survey research and sampling.* Asheboro, NC: Statistical Publishing Associates.

Hunter, J. E., & Schmidt, F. L. (2015). *Methods of meta-analysis: Correcting error and bias in research findings* (3rd ed.). Thousand Oaks, CA: Sage.

Wampold, B. E., & Imel, Z. E. (2015). *The great psychotherapy debate: Evidence for what makes psychotherapy work* (2nd ed.). Mahwah, NJ: Erlbaum.

8

Translating Research
Into Practice

H AVING NOW CRITICALLY APPRAISED THE RESEARCH
reports, you begin to translate the research into practice. You
become a critical consumer and interpreter of the research evidence as it applies to your clinical situation at hand. Beyond browsing the literature, your aim now involves using the information in
solving patient problems and in improving your care (Guyatt &
Rennie, 2002).

In this chapter, we will assist you in translating that research evidence for direct application to your patients. First, we address the
imperative of translational research and the stance of the reflective
practitioner. We help you translate the results of randomized clinical trials (RCTs) into practice by applying the CONSORT standards
(as graphically illustrated in Chapter 7) and working through the
CONSORT checklist. Next, we help you to consider potential harms
that might accrue to your patients in applying the research to them.
We also discuss the process of identifying discredited practices—
interventions that do not work—and reflect on how to proceed in the
face of inconsistent evidence. Finally, we provide a quick lesson in
applying clinical decision analysis by using decision trees to explore
choices at critical junctures.

Translational Research: Identifying What Works

Practitioners in the behavioral health and addiction field have increasingly become aware that the science-to-service or (lab) bench-to-bedside process runs along a two-way street. Basic scientists or clinical investigators provide practitioners with new tools; practitioners often make novel observations about the nature and progression of disorders that stimulate additional investigations. Patient and family member reports of outcomes help close the feedback loop and generate more research ideas.

Perhaps the worst feeling experienced by a practitioner is the sense of helplessness when one lacks sufficient knowledge to alleviate a client's distress. Each year, more than 6 million adults and 3 million children in the United States experience debilitating symptoms at the termination of treatment (National Advisory Mental Health Council on Behavioral Science, 2000). Although advances in science and practice have improved treatment outcomes (Lambert & Ogles, 2004), a pressing need remains to develop more effective interventions for the many patients who do not respond to current treatments (Hannan et al., 2005).

In an effort to promote development of innovative treatments, the National Institute of Mental Health (NIMH) has placed strong emphasis on **translational research**. The NIMH definition states, "Translational research in the behavioral and social sciences addresses how basic behavioral processes inform the diagnosis, prevention, treatment, and delivery of services for mental illness, and, conversely, how knowledge of mental illness increases our understanding of basic behavioral processes" (National Advisory Mental Health Council on Behavioral Science, 2000, p. iii). In other words, translational research deals with how best to move research evidence from scholarly journals to consulting rooms.

You can begin translating research evidence to your practice by considering significant methodological decisions made by the researchers whose work you read. Five methodological foci characterize successful programs of translational research: (1) time span, (2) scope of hypotheses, (3) dose adjustments, (4) determining contraindications, and (5) selection of patient population. Early-phase translational research usually begins with short time frames, addresses hypotheses with relatively narrow scope, delivers small doses of treatment, and closely monitors any potential for harm (contraindications). The defining features of translational research become clearly evident in the middle phases, when time lengthens, the scopes of hypotheses broaden, and doses of presumably active interventions increase in trials with low-risk patient populations. In later-phase translational research, larger, full-scale clinical trials begin to test the efficacy and effectiveness of interventions with diverse patient populations (Tashiro & Mortensen, 2006). Research in the middle and later phases can be translated into daily clinical practice.

Becoming a Reflective Practitioner

In critically appraising what you have found in your search of the research literature, we recommend the old German proverb "Zu glauben alles zu viel, nichts zu glauben ist nicht genug" (To believe everything is too much, to believe nothing is not enough).

Beginners tend to follow one of two error-prone paths. First, some give in to the pervasive temptation to prematurely dismiss or trash the research literature as "not like my patient" or "not compelling research." Rarely, if ever, will any single review or meta-analysis perfectly match your patient and context. We must assume that any piece of research suffers from imperfections, especially with respect to any direct translation from the laboratory to the consulting room. But will the data prove good enough to let us draw reasonable guidance? Second, other beginners succumb to the temptation to worship all publishable research and automatically apply it to their particular circumstances. Nonresearchers often find it difficult to appreciate the contextual and subjective limits of science. We must thoughtfully ask, can the research translate to my patient?

In seeking to integrate research into clinical practice, we adopt the notion of the *reflective practitioner* (Peterson, 1995). Frequently we find a tension between scientific rigor, on the one hand, and clinical relevance, on the other. This tension is frequently characterized as **efficacy research** versus **effectiveness research**. Researchers cannot easily control and randomize all important variables, such as empathy, therapeutic relationship, and patient comorbidity. However, practitioners need not fly off into an intuitive "never-never land." Reflection in action means drawing on past research and documented theory wherever pertinent research has occurred and well-tested theories exist. As Peterson (1995, p. 980) puts it, "Whenever high ground appears, we need to seize it, hold it, and work from it in the public benefit." The reflective, sophisticated practitioner will rely on empirical research when available and when relevant to a particular case. In the words of the APA Task Force on Evidence-Based Practice (2006, p. 285): "The treating psychologist determines the applicability of research conclusions to a particular patient. Individual patients may require decisions and interventions not directly addressed by the available research."

The task confronting the reflective practitioner consists of recognizing boundary conditions when deciding whether research (and if so, which research) applies to the current clinical situation. At least three key questions flow from this line of reasoning (Semple et al., 2005):

♦ Does the quality of the research pass muster (validity), as detailed in Chapters 5, 6, and 7?
♦ Does the research hold enough relevance to the current situation to warrant attempting to apply it?
♦ Does the research match my patient and context (**transportability**) closely enough?

In the hierarchy of research evidence, the results of RCTs and summaries/meta-analyses of multiple RCTs have traditionally emerged as the gold standard for informing evidence-based practices (EBPs). Thus, we concentrate on extrapolating from clinical trials to individual patients, with a focus on RCTs. As noted in Chapter 5, these studies come closest to allowing us to draw causal conclusions from data.

Evaluating Randomized Clinical Trials

Novices and nonresearchers sometimes have difficulty appreciating the subjectivity of science. An aphorism reminds us: Scientists are scientific about everything but their own science! Decisions about inclusion criteria, outcome measures, research designs, comparison groups, and the like can bias or even preordain results.

Consider the controversial example of the effectiveness of abstinence-only programs aimed at reducing youthful sexual activity, and thereby pregnancies and sexually transmitted diseases. Early studies suggested that abstinence-only programs proved effective in reducing early sexual activity. But later, well-controlled studies repeatedly found that children and adolescents enrolled in abstinence-only intervention programs had no greater likelihood of abstaining than did their control group counterparts. We need to just say "no!"—to bad science (Begley, 2007).

 Skill Exercise 8-1

Design your own psychotherapy outcome RCT with preordained results to your liking. Choose your hypotheses and specify inclusion criteria, outcome measures, comparison groups, and the like to set up your results to almost certainly support the hypotheses. Then, by contrast, design a psychotherapy outcome RCT for the same patients that would *not* favor preordained results and that would feature bona fide comparison groups and impartial inclusion criteria.

Undeniably, RCTs constitute an advance in healthcare as a means of determining treatment effects while controlling other factors that might affect patient outcomes. At the same time, significant mismatches exist between the evidence provided by RCTs and the needs of practitioners. Because many factors other than the treatment itself profoundly alter a patient's outcome, determining the best treatment (or assessment, prevention, etc.) for any particular patient in any given situation will differ fundamentally from determining which treatment proves best on average (Kent & Hayward, 2007). We do not mean to suggest that RCTs cannot inform our approach to individual patients but rather that they cannot alone determine our direction and should never shackle us.

Reporting a single number from an RCT, such as an effect size or an absolute risk reduction, gives the misleading impression that the treatment method alone accounted for the outcome. Such impressions ignore the interaction between the multifaceted method and the complex risk–benefit profile of a particular group of patients (Kent & Hayward, 2007). Even when RCT results yield no differentially beneficial effects, some patients may still benefit substantially from the treatment. Alternatively, a treatment that benefits many on average may prove ineffective for particular others. Some risks and benefits also go undetected in clinical trials, hidden because study designs mask individual differences.

Another concern arises from the fact that RCTs have evolved more recently, appear with less frequency, and use less rigorous methodologies in behavioral health and addictions than in biomedical research. The RCTs reported in behavioral journals tend to reflect more analytic weaknesses than those reported in medical journals, particularly with regard to specifying primary outcomes, analyzing intention to treat, randomizing all participants, and accounting for missing data (Spring et al., 2007). Simply put, RCTs in medical journals are generally more sophisticated and complete.

The international team of researchers known as the CONSORT (Consolidated Standards of Reporting Trials) group (Moher et al., 2001a, 2001b; Schulz et al., 2010) created reporting guidelines for RCTs. These guidelines have won wide endorsement in biomedical and behavioral journals and have increased standardization and transparency of reporting results. Many journals now recommend or require a CONSORT flow chart (see Figure 7.5). The CONSORT guidelines are a particular boon to those trying to evaluate and synthesize research reports. We summarize the 25 items of CONSORT's checklist for reporting an RCT in Table 8.1.

As you can see, compliance with the CONSORT standards enables the reader to draw significant translational implications. For example, readers can quickly gauge eligibility, inclusion, exclusion, and elimination criteria to assist them in assessing how closely the study sample matches particular patients. We can trace the sequence of participants through the study, evaluate the relevance and utility of the outcome measures, and even check for common adverse effects. Finally, the CONSORT standards specifically mandate that investigators address the generalizability of the findings. As we read through the flow chart and focus on the CONSORT criteria, we can imagine precisely how any of our particular patients might have wound their way through the study.

Many types of research designs (e.g., case series, harm analyses, epidemiological reports, field surveys) now have reporting guidelines. The

TABLE 8.1 Summary of CONSORT 2010 Checklist for Reporting a Randomized Trial

Paper section	Item	Description
Title and abstract	1	Identification as a randomized trial in the title; structured summary of trial design, methods, results, and conclusions
Background and objectives	2	Scientific background and explanation of rationale; specific objectives or hypotheses
Trial design	3	Description of study design, including changes to methods after the trial commenced
Participants	4	Eligibility criteria for participants; settings and locations where data were collected
Interventions	5	Interventions with sufficient details to allow replication; how and when treatments were actually administered
Outcomes	6	Completely defined primary and secondary outcome measures, including any changes to outcomes after the trial commenced
Sample size	7	How sample size was determined and, when applicable, explanation of any interim analyses and stopping rules
Randomization—sequence generation	8	Method used to generate the random allocation sequence, including details of any restrictions (e.g., blocking, stratification)
Randomization—allocation concealment	9	Mechanism used to implement the random allocation sequence (e.g., numbered containers), describing any steps to conceal the sequence until interventions were assigned
Randomization—implementation	10	Who generated the allocation sequence, who enrolled participants, and who assigned participants to their groups
Blinding (masking)	11	Whether or not participants, those administering the interventions, and those assessing the outcomes were blinded to group assignment. If done, how the success of blinding was evaluated

(continued)

TABLE 8.1 Summary of CONSORT 2010 Checklist for Reporting a Randomized Trial (Continued)

Paper section	Item	Description
Statistical methods	12	Statistical methods used to compare groups for primary outcome(s); methods for additional analyses, such as subgroup analyses and adjusted analyses
Participant flow	13	Flow of participants through study (a flow diagram); for each group, report the numbers of participants randomly assigned, received intended treatment, completed the study, and analyzed. Describe losses and deviations after randomization
Recruitment	14	Dates defining the periods of recruitment and follow-up; why trial ended or was stopped
Baseline data	15	Baseline demographic and clinical characteristics of each group
Numbers analyzed	16	Number of participants (denominator) in each group included in each analysis and whether the analysis was by original assigned groups
Outcomes and estimation	17	For each primary and secondary outcome, summarize results for each group and the estimated effect size and its precision (e.g., 95% confidence interval)
Ancillary analyses	18	Results of any other analyses performed, including subgroup analyses and adjusted analyses
Harms	19	All important harms or unintended effects in each group
Discussion—limitations	20	Trial limitations, including sources of potential bias, imprecision, and multiplicity of analyses
Discussion—generalizability	21	Report on generalizability (external validity, applicability) of the findings
Discussion—interpretation	22	Interpretation consistent with results, balancing benefits and harms, considering other relevant evidence
Registration	23	Registration number and name of trial
Protocol	24	Where full trial protocol can be accessed, if any
Funding	25	Sources of funding and other support; role of funders in the study

Note: Adapted from CONSORT at www.consort-statement.org/.

Equator Network (www.equator-network.org/reporting-guidelines/) has collected more than 290 of these reporting guidelines, including CONSORT's.

In addition to the CONSORT items (and other reporting guidelines), we suggest attending to a few other vital considerations when critically appraising RCTs and systematic reviews for behavioral health and substance abuse outcomes:

♦ What determined the salubrious effect reported? Consider the treatment method, practitioner characteristics, patient attributes, and the therapeutic relationship. Does the treatment method appear to receive credit properly due to the therapy relationship or individual practitioner?

♦ Can we safely assume that efficacious EBP assessments, treatments, and preventions validated on a homogeneous patient population will work equally well for other groups, particularly cultural, ethnic, or racial minority groups?

♦ Do the inclusion and exclusion criteria seem reasonable, or do they constrain validity by narrowing the study sample too much? In a meta-analysis of published outcome studies on three disorders, investigators estimated the average inclusion rates to be only 32% for depression, 36% for panic disorder, and 35% for generalized anxiety disorder (Westen & Morrison, 2001). The typical study excluded the majority of the individuals who sought treatment for one of these disorders.

♦ Should we feel concerned about publication bias? For example, does the journal or online resource have a peer review policy or a narrow theoretical perspective that might cause us concern?

♦ Can we feel confident about effect sizes? Do we find credible evidence of clinical significance in addition to statistical significance? (See Chapter 6 for explanation of effect size.)

♦ Do the outcome measures have relevance for the symptoms or concerns we seek to treat in our clients?

♦ Does the RCT use bona fide comparisons? The data show the treatment worked, but compared with what? For example, was a new treatment compared against an existing standard or treatment as usual (TAU) or against no treatment, a waiting list, or a sham control group of some sort? It is relatively easy to show that a treatment, any treatment, outperformed no treatment, but it is quite difficult to demonstrate that a treatment outperformed a bona fide alternative treatment (Wampold & Imel, 2015).

♦ Do the lead researchers have a theoretical allegiance that may have led to a bias in conducting the study or analyses? The researcher's allegiance has been shown to account for more than half of all purported outcome differences among psychotherapies (Luborsky et al., 1999).

♦ When a funding source is identified, did it likely bias the design, the implementation, or the reporting of the results? This can prove a particular concern in medication trials funded by drug companies or other sources with an agenda. For example, in the case of *Daubert v. Merrell Dow Pharmaceuticals, Inc.*, described in Chapter 10, a legal team tried to submit research from drug studies that were run chiefly to provide potential evidence for the litigation. Some corporate entities fund research with a requirement that they retain the right to block publication of the data if they so choose. Should we trust such research? Do such studies constitute dispassionate scientific evidence or subtle efforts to selectively market commercial products?

♦ Is the EBP under study the only one or the most effective one of its kind? Have the researchers ignored or overlooked important alternatives?

♦ What are the probabilities of relapse (see Witkiewitz & Marlatt, 2007)?

♦ Do the findings apply reasonably well to our particular treatment setting?

By asking yourself these questions as you read an RCT, you can avoid uncritical acceptance of relatively useless or misleading information while concentrating on the most generalizable components with the greatest relevance to the particular patient(s) of concern.

How Much Bias?

During our workshops and talks on EBP, challenging questions often come up about the multiple sources of bias in designing, implementing, and reporting the results of RCTs. Most practitioners know about the replicated and apparently ubiquitous effects of researchers' allegiance (Luborsky et al., 1999), explained above. But other potential biases can exert substantial impact on what people convey as the best available research evidence. Most of these biases become identifiable when researchers faithfully adhere to the CONSORT reporting standards.

Consider a handful of other biases and the evidence of their probable effects. One concerns the involvement of pharmaceutical companies in medication trials. A recent evaluation of 185 meta-analyses of antidepressant medication studies found that one third of the published articles were written by pharmaceutical industry employees. About 80% of the meta-analyses had some sort of industry tie, through either funding or conflicts of interest. Meta-analyses written by pharmaceutical industry employees were 22 times less likely to contain negative statements about a medication than those written by unaffiliated researchers (Jacobson, 2015). Sponsorship by the manufacturers of medical devices also led to more favorable results and conclusions than did sponsorship by other sources (Lundh et al., 2012). Bottom line: Remain wary of the clinical conclusions drawn in healthcare RCTs and meta-analyses written by authors employed by or affiliated with Big Pharma.

One hidden bias involves researchers exploring data in multiple ways before deciding which analyses provide the most favorable, and publishable, results. This **opportunistic bias** results in published findings that seem stronger and otherwise more supportive of researchers' theories than they would have seemed without the relentless data exploration. The magnitudes of opportunistic bias may often be as strong as those of the effects under investigation, leading to invalid conclusions (DeCoster et al., 2015). Authors do not typically report their exploratory statistical procedures, so this bias becomes almost impossible to detect by reading the final version of a research report. That's why the CONSORT guidelines urge authors to describe the results of all ancillary analyses—but few authors do so. In a related vein, sometimes authors report all analyses but emphasize only "significant" results in summarizing the study, leaving nonsignificant results buried in a multitude of tables.

A final potential bias covered here concerns the multiple methodological decisions in psychotherapy studies that stack the deck in the researchers' favor. Take the example of the reported advantage of research-supported treatments over treatment as usual (TAU) in the treatment of youths. The decisions included whether the TAU qualified as a bona fide therapy, whether all therapists received clinical supervision, and whether specialized training was provided only to the research-supported therapists. When controlling for these confounds, the reported advantages of the research-supported therapies over TAU became small and nearly always statistically and clinically nonsignificant (Spielmans et al., 2010). Lesson learned: Always consider the structural, training, and supervision equivalence of compared treatments.

Extrascientific biases occur in all human endeavors (as detailed in Chapter 10), and behavioral health research is no exception. Indeed, there is every reason to believe that the biases discussed above as well as others operate in all research designs, probably even more so in uncontrolled case studies and naturalistic pre–post designs than in RCTs. But let's not overreact and discredit all scientific research. Our response to the question (and challenge) of biases in RCTs holds that while they certainly exist, research acts as a self-correcting process, and steps exist to identify and reduce the impact of these biases. The evidence-based practitioner must remain an informed and skeptical consumer.

 Skill Exercise 8-2

Search the unfiltered literature (through PsycINFO or PubMed) for a recent RCT conducted on one of your favorite clinical methods or diagnostic populations. Read the results with an eye toward detecting the potential biases just explicated. Which biases did you detect? Which biases did you suspect but could not verify owing to insufficient information? Which potential biases were specifically controlled for or explained in the results?

Potential Harm

Recall the old saw "The operation was a success, but the patient died." Even with the best of evidence-based care, not everyone gets better. When translating research into practice, pay particular attention to the percentage of patients in RCTs who demonstrate no change or who deteriorate. Heed the Hippocratic oath: "First, do no harm."

Approximately 5–10% of patients will deteriorate during the course of behavioral health and addiction treatment (Lambert & Ogles, 2004), and another 20–25% of patients will fail to respond to the treatment (Lambert, 2010). Note that these figures apply *during* the course of treatment, not necessarily *because* of the treatment. Nonetheless, a small portion of patients will experience harm, and a larger proportion will experience no meaningful improvement as a result of treatment, and we must consider these phenomena when translating research into clinical practice. What is the likelihood that this particular patient may suffer harm? What price is the cure?

One way to reduce the risk of patient harm or deterioration during the course of treatment involves conducting a **decision analysis**, a process we discuss later in this chapter. Simpler processes involve **cost–benefit analysis** and **risk–benefit analysis**. The primary difference between these two involves whether one focuses on all risks or only economic hazards.

Economic costs include the total dollar amount paid to a clinician or agency for services, whether the patient pays the full fee out of pocket, covers a copayment charge, or is covered by health insurance. Additional fiscal components include incidental costs (e.g., for prescription drugs, transportation, and child care) and opportunity costs (e.g., time lost from work or school). Of course, mental disorders and substance abuse have economic costs of their own (lost productivity, disability payments, etc.). Some treatments will prove more costly than others, and the costs will be borne by different parties.

Annique's health insurance covers most of the cost of her psychotherapy and medications. Depending on her coverage, some medications may cost her significantly more than others; some practitioners may not qualify as in-network reimbursable under her plan; the number of sessions and types of services may fall under managed-care restrictions; and her preferred treatment options (or the most effective EBP practitioners) may not fall under her coverage mandates. On the other hand, Annique's health insurance may favor EBP and professionals known to use such approaches. The company may offer her incentives (e.g., lower copayments) to use such clinicians or may require clinicians to certify that they use EBPs.

Francesco has neither employment nor insurance, so he must rely on state services for the uninsured or take advantage of agencies offering low fees or pro bono services. In that sense, the rest of society contributes (via taxes or higher fees) to cover the cost of any services he receives. Different EBPs pose different costs and different potential benefits for him, but much relies on his preferences and motivations. For example, outpatient treatment with cognitive–behavior therapy focused on his anxiety and delivered through a community agency might help him, but his alcohol abuse might erode those gains. An intensive inpatient program coupling cognitive–behavior therapy with state-of-the-art substance abuse treatment might prove more effective or have a more enduring effect but lie beyond his (and society's) financial means. Whether he will have access to EBPs remains unclear, but the costs rise steeply if he is not treated. If his anxiety leads to continued unemployment or his alcohol abuse leads to liver disease requiring medical attention or results in incarceration for acts he committed while intoxicated, considerable public costs accrue.

From a purely economic perspective, patients and society will more likely than not benefit from the ready availability of EBPs in the long run, because the average patient will improve and become more productive (or cease being an economic drain) more quickly. Making such services available, however, may prove more expensive in the short run (e.g., because of the costs of providing necessary education and training to practitioners and ensuring patient access to same).

In a risk–benefit analysis, cost becomes but one factor. Other hazards include side effects of biological treatments (e.g., medication, electroshock, deep brain stimulation) and risks associated with treatment (e.g., diagnostic errors, misapplied techniques, therapist negligence). In general, properly applied EBPs tend by their very nature to minimize risk when used appropriately (see the discussion of professional liability in Chapter 10).

The Dark Side: Identifying What Does *Not* Work

The President's New Freedom Commission on Mental Health in 2003 called attention to both the *underuse* of evidence-based treatments and the *overuse* of treatments for which no favorable empirical evidence exists. Practitioners are encouraged to simultaneously use EBPs to promote what *does* work and avoid discredited practices to eradicate what does *not* work. In other words, translational research can be prescriptive as well as proscriptive.

Specific assessments, treatments, and prevention programs that have not been subjected to systematic empirical testing cannot be assumed to be either effective or ineffective; they are simply untested to date. The absence of evidence, we must recall, is not evidence of absence.

But there exist assessment, treatment, and prevention practices that are discredited, even harmful. **Discredited practices** are those unable to consistently generate treatment outcomes (in the case of interventions) or valid data (in the case of assessments) beyond those obtained by the passage of time alone, expectancy, base rates, or credible placebos. While the term *discredited* subsumes ineffective and detrimental interventions, it forms a broader and more inclusive characterization (Norcross et al., 2006b).

In three recent Delphi polls, we asked respected experts to rate the degree to which various practices in mental health and addictions were discredited (Koocher et al., 2014; Norcross et al., 2006b, 2010). Box 8.1 summarizes expert consensus on the most discredited treatments and tests. These are generally to be avoided. As one example, consider the research on critical incident stress debriefing (CISD). The RCTs show that CISD heightens risk for post-traumatic stress symptoms in some individuals (Lilienfeld, 2007).

Another potentially harmful set of interventions, described as *sexual orientation conversion* or *reparative therapies*, purport to resolve unwanted same-sex attraction via verbal psychotherapy laced with a significant religious overlay. Some clients uncomfortable with same-sex attraction have sought and benefited from psychotherapy, but rigorous empirical studies fail to show that conversion therapies work (Greene et al., 2007; Schneider et al., 2002). We must therefore ask whether offering such treatments comports with the therapist's ethical responsibility and consumer welfare. Both professional organizations and some state legislatures have enacted strictures against such conversion therapies.

Box 8.1 Expert Consensus on Discredited Practices in Mental Health and Addictions

Top 10 discredited mental health treatments for adults

1. Angel therapy for treatment of mental/behavioral disorders
2. Use of pyramids for restoration of energy
3. Orgone therapy (use of orgone energy accumulator) for treatment of mental/behavioral disorders
4. Crystal healing for treatment of mental/behavioral disorders
5. Past-life therapy for treatment of mental/behavioral disorders
6. Future-lives therapy for treatment of mental/behavioral disorders
7. Treatments of post-traumatic stress disorder caused by alien abduction
8. Rebirthing therapies for treatment of mental/behavioral disorders
9. Color therapy for treatment of mental/behavioral disorders
10. Primal scream therapy for treatment of mental/behavioral disorders

Top 10 discredited mental health treatments for children

1. Magnet therapy for treatment of child psychopathology
2. Past-life regression therapy for treatment of child psychopathology
3. Rebirthing therapy for treatment of child psychopathology
4. Crystal healing for treatment of child psychopathology
5. Bio-Ching for treatment of child psychopathology
6. JoyTouch for treatment of child psychopathology
7. Kirlian therapy for treatment of child psychopathology
8. Penduluming for treatment of child psychopathology
9. Withholding food or water for treatment of child psychopathology
10. Aura therapy for treatment of child psychopathology

Top 10 discredited substance abuse treatments

1. Electrical stimulation of the head for alcohol dependence
2. Past-life therapy for drug addictions and for alcohol dependence[a]
3. Metronidazole for alcohol dependence
4. Electric shock for alcohol dependence
5. Psychedelic medication for alcohol dependence
6. Ultrarapid opioid detoxification under anesthesia for alcohol dependence
7. Neurolinguistic programming for drug and alcohol dependence
8. Scared Straight for prevention of alcohol dependence and for prevention of drug abuse[a]
9. Stimulant medications for alcohol dependence
10. DARE (Drug Abuse Resistance Education) programs for prevention of substance abuse

Top 10 discredited psychological tests

1. Lüscher Color Test for personality assessment
2. Szondi Test for personality assessment
3. Handwriting analysis (graphology) for personality assessment
4. Bender Visual Motor Gestalt Test for assessment of neuropsychological impairment
5. Enneagrams for personality assessment
6. Lowenfeld Mosaic Test for personality assessment
7. Bender Visual Motor Gestalt Test for personality assessment
8. Anatomically detailed dolls or puppets for determining if a child was sexually abused
9. Blacky Pictures Test for personality assessment
10. Hand Test for personality assessment

[a] These practices rated as discredited for both alcohol and drug abuse in separate items.
Adapted from Koocher et al. (2014); Norcross et al. (2006b, 2010).

Skill Exercise 8-3

Choose a potentially discredited method from the lists provided or from your own experience and readings. Find a published data-based article advocating the method and review it using the CONSORT criteria or other strategies suggested in this chapter. Do the results of your analysis surprise you?

The Muddle: Inconsistent Research Evidence

Evidence-based practice is reasonably easy when the research evidence is unmistakably clear: Do not engage in practices that are consensually regarded as discredited or detrimental, and consider employing those practices that receive unequivocal support in the research literature. Alas, clinical reality is rarely so accommodating. Many times the research evidence says "maybe" or "perhaps" because of inconsistent results.

Sometimes that inconsistency can be resolved by moderator analyses. An example comes from the psychotherapy literature. For decades, researchers searched for—and expected to find—a positive effect on treatment from matching the sex of the patient to the sex of the clinician (woman to woman, man to man). That search proved unsuccessful; the research did not support the expected effect (Sue & Lam, 2002). But then we discovered that automatically matching the therapy dyads was sexually and culturally insensitive; the positive effect emerged only when the patient expressed a strong preference for a therapist of a particular sex (Swift et al., 2011). In those instances, preferences acted as a moderator, and the inconsistent research findings became explainable.

But more times than not, we cannot explain away inconsistency in the research evidence by conducting additional analyses or considering another variable. In such instances, what should a well-intentioned clinician do when confronted with between-study inconsistencies on what works?

Following the lead of others (e.g., De Los Reyes & Kazdin, 2008), we recommend examining the systematic reviews and meta-analyses for the preponderance of evidence. That examination should result in one of several broad categories of evidence for effectiveness, as displayed in Table 8.2. *Effectiveness* in this context refers to whether the treatment, prevention, assessment, or other clinical service has been shown to prove valuable or effective in the extant research. Note that the criteria for effectiveness depend not only on the percentage of supportive studies but also on whether there is a preponderance of evidence from different outcome measures (e.g., self-report of symptoms, diagnostic interviews, clinician judgments) and analytic methods (e.g., tests of mean differences, tests of diagnostic status). In this way, one can look simultaneously both at the big clinical

TABLE 8.2 Preponderance of Research Evidence for Intervention Effectiveness

Category	Criteria
Best evidence for effectiveness	At least 80% of the published findings from three or more outcome measures and analytic methods show effectiveness. No clear measure- or method-specific pattern of findings emerges.
Evidence for probable effectiveness	More than 50% of the published findings from three or more outcome measures and analytic methods show effectiveness. There is no clear measure- or method-specific pattern of findings.
Limited and inconclusive evidence of effectiveness	No more than 50% of the published findings from three or more outcome measures and analytic methods show effectiveness. The differences scatter across measures and methods.
No evidence of effectiveness	No published findings report significant effectiveness. No conclusive evidence exists.
Evidence for measure- or method-specific effectiveness	Differences in effectiveness appear on 80% or more of specific outcome measure(s) or analytic method(s). The evidence suggests that the intervention may prove effective when assessed with/applied to those measure(s), method(s), or both.

Note: Adapted from and inspired by De Los Reyes & Kazdin (2008).

picture—what percentage of studies report effectiveness—and at several research features—what between-study patterns reveal.

Consider the case of Annique and her major depressive disorder and dependent personality disorder. There are at least 100 published RCTs on psychotherapy and pharmacotherapy for the treatment of depression and dozens of meta-analytic summaries of that research evidence. But for dependent personality disorder, one finds a muddle. Precious few RCTs on the treatment of personality disorders exist (except for borderline personality disorder), so we are left with only a couple of controlled efficacy studies and several naturalistic effectiveness studies. In circumstances like these, the evidence-based practitioner will gratefully assimilate the few extant controlled studies and tentatively accept several supportive naturalistic studies as providing "limited evidence" or evidence of "probable effectiveness." Some research trumps no research in such cases.

The broad guidelines in Table 8.2 for interpreting inconsistent research evidence can help practitioners navigate the muddle. A consistent framework in approaching mixed conclusions will probably increase the reliability and validity of clinician conclusions (De Los Reyes & Kazdin, 2008). Sometimes relying on available research evidence, albeit ambiguous, works better than using none at all.

Clinical Decision Analysis

Traditional decision analysis texts often attempt to teach would-be decision makers about the influence of probabilities and preferences using the hypothetical "stranded on a desert island without food or water" scenario. The instructor tells the students to assume that a bottle washes ashore, they uncork it, and in so doing they release a genie who offers a food reward for releasing him, but with a catch: The stranded hungry person must play a game of chance with three potential outcomes: a 95% chance of winning a moldy, stale loaf of bread and glass of tepid water; a 50% chance of winning a sandwich and beverage of choice; or a 25% chance of winning a sumptuous seven-course meal imported from a five-star restaurant. Which would you choose? The ultrarational survivalist would pick the nearly certain win of bread and water. But wait: Perhaps the castaway only just arrived on the island, does not feel particularly hungry, has an intense mold aversion, and anticipates rescue in the near future. In those circumstances, the other options become more appealing. The intrinsic message: People's preferences, beliefs, and perceptions of probable outcomes exert a powerful influence on their decisions.

When making clinical decisions about behavioral health treatment, clinicians often behave in a similar fashion—relying on internalized preferences, theoretical orientations, and probability estimates. They weigh preferences and perceived probabilities in deciding what course to follow. Sometimes they will decline a highly effective treatment because they perceive the cost as too high or the value as too low. Sometimes the costs considered are economic (price); other times the decision may flow from perceptions about quality of life or likely outcome.

Let us walk through a decision analysis for a particular patient to illustrate in somewhat simplified form the stepwise process of translating research into practice. Figure 8.1 displays a simplified decision tree for Jonathon's diagnosis. The referral information from the school psychologist informs us that "Psychological testing, behavioral observations, and record review supported a diagnosis of ADHD (mixed type) and mild-to-moderate oppositional defiant disorder (ODD) accompanied by family tensions." As good clinicians we cannot assume the accuracy of the referring diagnosis and should evaluate Jonathon's status as a precursor to formulating a treatment plan.

Figure 8.1 shows the array of potential diagnoses that could account for Jonathon's problems. Your review of the literature suggests that the probability of an accurate ADHD diagnosis in boys Jonathon's age is approximately 4–8%; thus we might consider assigning a probability value of 6% at the decision choice point for making an ADHD diagnosis, indicated by the double line. If we simply guess that the ADHD diagnosis applies, we will have a 6% shot at accurate diagnosis by chance alone. Similarly, a valid diagnosis of Tourette syndrome would prove accurate only 0.03% of the time, based on epidemiological rates alone. We know that Jonathon's asthma medication, albuterol, can cause nervousness, irritability, restlessness, and sleep problems, but the incidence studies of side effects become difficult to interpret because of dosing differences and the small numbers of child participants in drug company studies. Published incidence data range from 3% to 20% for "moderate level" symptoms.

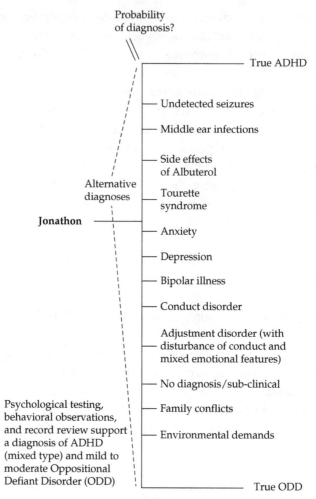

FIGURE 8.1 Simplified decision tree for diagnosis of Jonathon.

In this case, knowledge of **epidemiology** can guide us in asking the right questions. For example, do Jonathon's difficulties increase on days when he needs to use his asthma inhaler? Has his physician tried other asthma medications that might reduce physiological correlates of agitation? Such data can also help us to eliminate low-incidence conditions such as Tourette syndrome, especially if Jonathon's symptoms do not seem fully congruent with them (e.g., no reports of tics or coprolalia). While the incidence-related probabilities offer a degree of guidance, we know (and suspect) that Jonathon's behavior difficulties most likely arise from an interaction of multiple causes.

We know that the reliability of assigning diagnoses suffers from many shortcomings, particularly in childhood. Research generally finds poor reliability among different diagnostic methods and different diagnosticians. One set of researchers (Lewczy et al., 2003), for example, studied agreement between diagnoses for 240 youths generated through parent and youth interviews with the structured Diagnostic Interview Schedule for Children (DISC) and diagnoses assigned by clinicians in community-based practice settings. The agreement between the two assessment methods proved weak, with coefficients of agreement κ (kappa) ranging from −.04 for anxiety disorders to .22 for ADHD. Such discrepancies raise grave concerns about reliability of diagnoses and assessment measures among children (Hoagwood, 2002).

We cannot be certain that Jonathon actually suffers from ADHD or ODD, but as clinicians we must make decisions. Researchers can respond to uncertainty with abstraction and curiosity; however, practitioners must resolve uncertainty through action (Greer, 1994). We must make diagnostic and treatment decisions on the basis of the best research at hand.

This necessity takes us to Figure 8.2, representing a simplified decision tree for treating Jonathon. For this tree we assume that we have eliminated all diagnoses other than ADHD and ODD. For each of those two disorders we show branches for both psychosocial and pharmacological treatments. Following one set of dashed lines, we could assign probabilities of beneficial response to each treatment based on published research and our confidence in those results. Note, however, the other dashed lines, at the points where the psychosocial and pharmacological options branch off, indicating the role of patient characteristics, cultures, and preferences. We know that these factors are all critical in determining the choice of treatment (see Chapter 9).

We also have learned from the school psychologist that "Jonathon's father firmly resists any psychotropic medication at this time" and that "both parents are genuinely concerned about Jonathon and willing to participate in a few family meetings, but their demanding work schedules and marital conflicts prevent extensive outpatient treatment." If we could convince Jonathon's father to allow a trial of stimulant medication, the next set of choices would involve a medication consultation to choose among the drugs with

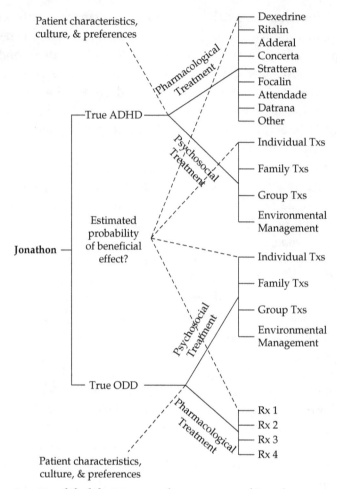

FIGURE 8.2 Simplified decision tree for treatment of Jonathon.

a record of documented success in treating ADHD. In making the choice we would have to consider the pluses and minuses of specific drug actions, side effects, interactions with Jonathon's other medication, and dosing (e.g., short acting vs. sustained release, oral delivery vs. transdermal patch).

In one sense, the father's reluctance to try additional medication could help if the ODD diagnosis proved more appropriate than ADHD. Although some prescribers have readily used atypical antipsychotic or other medications to treat ODD, these would all qualify as off-label uses under Food and Drug Administration regulations.

Treating ODD with medication has practically no research support; thus the risks far outweigh any benefit.

Given the record of family and school problems, however, any good child clinician will know that Jonathon will need more treatment than simply medication. The parents have demands on their time and a conflictual relationship, so the clinician will probably conclude that any intervention with the family will need a tight focus and prompt reinforcement for the frustrated parents. The clinician may want to use the well-established method of parent management training, but she knows that she has little chance of getting them to sign on for multiple sessions. She may find herself selecting those components of an EBP that she can adapt quickly in the hope of engaging the parents and helping them get a handle on the difficulties with their son. She will also have to make a clinical decision about whether she will have the best results delivering the parent training to the parents as a couple or as individuals, given the tensions between them. She will have a number of solid EBPs to guide her but most likely will not be able to deliver any of them to this family in the way that the protocol authors conducted the underlying research.

Interestingly, the clinician would face a similar pattern of decisions if she determined ODD to be the primary diagnosis. The target behaviors she would focus on would differ—managing temper outbursts for ODD as opposed to increasing planful behaviors with ADHD—but the need to help the parents and school with behavior management would not change.

This walk through the diagnostic and therapeutic decision trees for Jonathon demonstrates the process of translating published research into clinical practice. The next step in EBP entails integrating the patient and clinician with the research, which is our goal in the next chapter.

Key Terms

cost–benefit analysis
decision analysis
discredited practices
effectiveness research
efficacy research

epidemiology
opportunistic bias
risk–benefit analysis
translational research
transportability

Recommended Readings and Websites

Calculating risks of harm, jamaevidence.mhmedical.com/Calculator.aspx and www.cmaj.ca/cgi/content/full/171/4/353

CONSORT, www.consort-statement.org

De Los Reyes, A., & Kazdin, A. E. (2008). When the evidence says, "Yes, no, and maybe so." Attending to and interpreting inconsistent findings among evidence-based interventions. *Current Directions in Psychological Science, 17,* 47–51.

Figueira, J., Greco, S., & Ehrgott, M. (Eds.). (2005). *Multiple criteria decision analysis: State of the art surveys.* New York, NY: Springer.

Gambrill, E. (2012). *Critical thinking in clinical practice: Improving the quality of judgments and decisions* (3rd ed.). Hoboken, NJ: Wiley.

Lambert, M. J. (2010). *Prevention of treatment failure: The use of measuring, monitoring, and feedback in clinical practice.* Washington, DC: American Psychological Association.

Magnavita, J. J. (Ed.). (2016). *Clinical decision-making in mental health practice.* Washington, DC: American Psychological Association.

Petitti, D. B. (2000). *Meta-analysis, decision analysis, and cost-effectiveness: Methods for quantitative synthesis in medicine* (2nd ed.). New York, NY: Oxford University Press.

President's New Freedom Commission on Mental Health. (2003). store.samhsa.gov/shin/content/SMA03-3831/SMA03-3831.pdf

9

Integrating the Patient and the Clinician With the Research

Y OU HAVE ASKED A SPECIFIC CLINICAL QUESTION, accessed the research literature, appraised that research, and, as illustrated in the last chapter, begun to translate it into clinical practice. Now we advance to the necessary and core skill of integrating the best available research with the two other pillars of evidence-based practice (EBP): the clinician's expertise and the patient's characteristics.

A fundamental premise of EBP holds that research alone will never suffice to make a clinical decision (Guyatt & Rennie, 2002). Indeed, the simple extrapolation of controlled research to practice does *not* qualify as EBP. Such a linear approach lacks clinical sophistication, sensitivity, and real-world application. Clinicians understandably rail against such naiveté and deride it as untenable "cookbook practice."

In practice, determining the optimal plan for a given patient constitutes a recursive process. After asking, "What does the research tell us?" we must always inquire: "What does the patient want? What is available and realistic? What fits this context? What about the cost–benefit ratio?" and a host of related questions. Then we ask, "Given these circumstances and this context, what does the research tell us now?" And so on, until we secure a seamless blend, a practical integration of best research, clinical expertise, and patient values.

In the words of George Eliot (the pen name of Mary Ann Evans) from the novel *The Mill on the Floss*, "we have no master-key that will fit all cases." We must make clinical decisions, like Eliot's moral decisions, by "exerting patience, discrimination, and impartiality" and an insight earned "from a life vivid and intense enough to have created a wide, fellow feeling with all that is human."

Yet, the integration of the three pillars of EBP remains the least developed (or most neglected) of the EBP skills. Proponents of evidence-based medicine tend to minimize this step; in fact, many equate it with translating the research. Apart from the literature on clinicians' decision-making (e.g., Garb, 1998; Magnavita, 2016), only a handful of empirical studies have examined clinical decision-making about behavioral and addiction treatments (Chambless & Crits-Christoph, 2005). As practitioners, we must acknowledge a dearth of EBPs about decision-making in realistic, complex situations. Until we possess better research, we depend upon generalizations from the extant, limited research and clinical expertise.

In a given case, we will need to make dozens of minidecisions, and there will never be empirical research to guide all of them. We cannot possibly expect that every practitioner's action will flow from research data (Chambless & Crits-Christoph, 2005). There remain many problem constellations and clinical situations for which empirical data are sparse. In such instances, clinicians must use their clinical expertise and the best available research evidence to develop coherent, realistic treatment strategies (APA Task Force on Evidence-Based Practice, 2006).

Pernicious Myths About Evidence-Based Practice

A core obstacle to practitioner acceptance and implementation of EBP stems from pervasive misunderstanding of its process and purpose. Let's correct the record here and now. We frequently encounter the following pernicious myths in our talks and workshops:

1. *EBP equates to a defined list of approved interventions.* No; EBP is a process. It consists of sequential skills (AAA TIE): *A*sking a specific clinical question; *A*ccessing the best available research; *A*ppraising that research evidence critically; *T*ranslating that

research into practice with a particular patient; *I*ntegrating the clinician's expertise and the patient's characteristics, culture, and preferences with the research; and *E*valuating the effectiveness of the entire process. A process, not a list, ultimately determined by the practitioner.

2. *Research alone determines what is EBP.* No, no, no! Research alone would constitute "research supported" or "empirically validated" practice but never EBP. To be sure, EBP begins with research, but it does not end there. Evidence-based practice requires the involvement of the patient and the clinician; otherwise, by definition, it cannot call itself EBP. Research is a necessary but never a sufficient component of EBP.

3. *Research-supported treatment means the "best" treatment.* Nope. What qualifies as "best" is multiply determined by the research, the patient, and the clinician. A slippery slope occurs when a clinical service has research support but its proponents tout it as the best treatment. Sadly, this sleight of hand routinely appears in publications, websites, and conversations.

4. *If a treatment has no RCTs for a particular disorder, we should not use it.* Yikes! Back to Logic 101: The absence of an RCT does *not* mean evidence of absence. "Untested in an RCT" must never be interpreted as equivalent to "ineffective." Absence of an RCT means just that: The treatment may be highly effective, mildly effective, or not effective at all. Research evidence other than RCTs counts as evidence. And research evidence is only one of the three essential components of EBP.

5. *The first in wins the race.* Evidence-based practice is not a speed race, but a power race. Cognitive–behavioral therapies and select medications rightfully deserve recognition as the first to establish solid research support of their efficacy. But appearing first does not mean demonstrating more effectiveness. Case in point: Cognitive therapy and antidepressants were among the first approaches tested in RCTs for unipolar depression, but we now know that at least half a dozen psychotherapies (e.g., interpersonal therapy, behavioral activation, and emotion-focused therapy) work equally well.

6. *What is frequently funded and researched in RCTs proves the most powerful elements.* Sadly, this is often not the case. As we will explain below, federal research grants favor the "medical–pharmaceutical model" in which discrete methods and medications

serve as the independent variables of interest. This is true despite decades of research showing that patient contributions, the therapeutic relationship, and individual-therapist effects are as potent, and probably more potent, than the particular treatment method (Lambert, 2013; Norcross, 2011; Wampold & Imel, 2015).

The net result of these myths among practitioners is confusion, anger, and avoidance (Wampold & Bhati, 2004). But when properly and inclusively defined, the process of EBP is welcomed. Of course, practitioners want to be informed by the best available research, and, of course, they want the best for their patients. And they desire to remain skilled and effective. Correctly identified, EBP proves a win-win-win-win for patients, practitioners, professions, and the populace.

Enlarging Decision-Making

Blending clinical expertise and patient characteristics, culture, and preferences with the research evidence will necessarily broaden our decision-making. In biomedicine, the prevalent model of treatment tends toward

Interventions → operate on patient's disease → to produce effects

The traditional medical–pharmaceutical model assumes that the curative power rests primarily with the method or intervention; that is, the relationship is hierarchically structured, with the provider serving as the expert, and the patient's role is to comply and participate as "prescribed" (Bohart, 2005).

In behavioral health and addiction practice, by contrast, the psychosocial model anticipates a more comprehensive and bidirectional process:

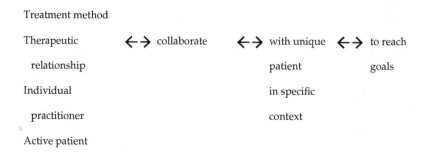

Treatment method			
Therapeutic	←→ collaborate	←→ with unique	←→ to reach
relationship		patient	goals
Individual		in specific	
practitioner		context	
Active patient			

The psychosocial model assumes that the curative power rests not only with the treatment method but also within the therapeutic relationship, the person of the practitioner, and the active client. Further, the treatment relationship works through collaboration, empathy, and support/validation. We filter and focus all decisions through the lens of the patient's characteristics, values, and culture. The client collaborates, remains informed, and works hard to participate and self-heal.

The psychosocial model requires us to abandon a parental stance and a passive image of patients and move toward a more collaborative stance and an active image of clients. The psychosocial model likewise rejects monocultural, one-size-fits-all treatments for a particular diagnosis in favor of culturally informed, individually tailored treatment plans. This chapter adopts as its template the psychosocial model, championed by behavioral health and addiction professionals for decades.

Clinical Expertise

Clinical expertise allows us to integrate the best research evidence with clinical data (e.g., information about the patient obtained over the course of treatment) in the context of **patient characteristics, culture, and preferences** to deliver services that have a high probability of achieving the goals of treatment (APA Task Force on Evidence-Based Practice, 2006). This description sounds accurate, but it raises the question of what exactly constitutes clinical expertise.

Let us begin by defining what does *not* qualify as clinical expertise. Clinical expertise does not refer to extraordinary performance that might characterize an elite group (e.g., the top 2%) of clinicians. (As an aside, the concept of rating someone a "top 2% clinician" ignores the obvious fact that no single clinician, regardless of wisdom, skill, and sophistication, will qualify as equally adept with every potential patient. It refers instead to skills expected of all well-trained behavioral health professionals.) Nor should we equate clinical expertise with clinical experience (Collins et al., 2007). Although clinical experience is required to develop clinical expertise, and ongoing clinical experience can enhance it, clinical expertise is a far more complicated and inclusive construct. Nor can we simply equate clinical expertise with theoretical orientation. Certainly, we expect clinical know-how to flow from a (testable) theory of psychopathology and behavior change. However, clinical expertise transcends the shackles of a single theoretical orientation to embrace specific, transtheoretical skills.

As the APA Task Force on Evidence-Based Practices (2006, p. 276) put it, clinical expertise

> encompasses a number of competencies that promote positive therapeutic outcomes. These competencies include a) conducting assessments and developing diagnostic judgments, systematic case formulations, and treatment plans; b) making clinical decisions, implementing treatments, and monitoring patient progress; c) possessing and using interpersonal expertise, including the formation of therapeutic alliances; d) continuing to self-reflect and acquire professional skills; e) evaluating and using research evidence in both basic and applied psychological science; f) understanding the influence of individual, cultural, and contextual differences on treatment; g) seeking available resources (e.g., consultation, adjunctive or alternative services) as needed; and h) having a cogent rationale for clinical strategies. Expertise develops from clinical and scientific training, theoretical understanding, experience, self-reflection, knowledge of current research, and continuing education and training.

Here, we shall punctuate just four of these competencies as they relate specifically to integrating the patient and the clinician with the research. First, clinical expertise includes a *scientific attitude* toward clinical work, characterized by openness to data, generation and testing of clinical hypotheses, and a commitment to not let theoretical preconceptions override clinical or research data. Second, clinical expertise entails the *skillful and flexible* delivery of treatment. Skill and flexibility require proficiency in delivering interventions and the ability to adapt the treatment to the particular case. Flexibility manifests in tact, timing, pacing, and framing of interventions such that an effective balance is struck between consistency of interventions and responsiveness to patient feedback. Third, clinical expertise does not end with determining an initial treatment plan; it entails *monitoring patient progress* (and changes in the patient's circumstances, such as job loss or major illness) that may suggest the need to adjust services. Should progress prove insufficient, the clinician considers alternative diagnoses and formulations, consultation, supervision, or referral. Fourth, clinical expertise requires an *awareness of the individual, social, and cultural context* of the patient. Such cultural sensitivity allows clinicians to adapt interventions and to construct a therapeutic milieu that respects the patient's worldview, values, and preferences.

Patient Characteristics, Cultures, and Preferences

The quality of medicine in the United States is exceptional in some categories, but dismal in others. Compared with other countries, the United States ranks poorly in coordinating the care of chronically ill patients, in meeting patient preferences, and in providing culture-sensitive services (World Health Organization, 2011). In other words, conventional medicine has not taken seriously patient characteristics, cultures, and preferences.

Behavioral health and substance abuse services prove most effective when responsive to the individual patient's specific problems, strengths, personality, sociocultural context, and preferences. In fact, many patient characteristics, such as functional status, readiness to change, and level of social support, have a documented relationship to therapeutic outcomes (see Norcross, 2011, for reviews).

The APA Task Force on Evidence-Based Practice (2006) described several important patient characteristics to consider in forming a treatment relationship and in implementing specific interventions. These include

- variations in presenting problems or disorders, etiology, and comorbid syndromes;
- chronological age, developmental status, developmental history, and life stage;
- sociocultural factors, including gender, gender identity, ethnicity, race, social class, religion, disability status, and sexual orientation;
- environmental context (e.g., institutional racism or health-care disparities) and stressors (e.g., unemployment or major life events); and
- personal preferences and values related to treatment (e.g., goals, beliefs, worldviews, and treatment expectations).

The explicit enumeration and delicate balancing of these multiple patient considerations bring underlying value judgments into bold relief (Guyatt & Rennie, 2002). Whose values do we see reflected in treatment decisions? Researchers'? Practitioners'? Patients'? Insurers'? And do we find those values (and their sources) explicitly articulated?

Many treatment guidelines, in particular, possess implicit values derived from the authors. For example, the outcomes of interest typically focus almost exclusively on symptom reduction (as opposed to, for example, increases in joy or insight), and the independent variables are typically treatment methods that can be controlled and randomized (as opposed to, say, a strong therapeutic relationship). In addition, most investigators study the performance of graduate students or licensed healthcare professionals (as opposed to, for example, indigenous healers or spiritual counselors). The investigators implicitly assume that one should always treat the disorders (e.g., as opposed to accepting diversity in functioning) and that treatments should continue until maximum benefit is achieved (as opposed to, for example, accepting an outcome as "good enough" or taking into account cost considerations). We rarely hear patient/consumer voices in the writing of treatment guidelines or compiling of research reviews.

We cannot anticipate the hundreds of patient considerations that potentially enter into the decision-making mix, but we have repeatedly noted several reality constraints that intrude on the process:

♦ *Readiness to change.* Only a minority of behavioral health and substance abuse patients enter treatment highly motivated and ready to immediately change their behavior (Prochaska et al., 2005). Instead, most patients enter treatment minimizing their problems, ambivalent about change, or merely contemplating taking action.

♦ *Acceptability.* Not all patients (or patient groups) will find the research-recommended intervention acceptable. Preference relates to what the patient desires; acceptability relates to what the patient finds minimally suitable.

♦ *Availability.* Access to the service (e.g., assessment, prevention, treatment) must exist locally and be affordable and available to the patient. Those individuals most in need of behavioral health and addiction treatment are frequently those who confront the most barriers to it. State-of-the-art, expensive services remain unavailable to many impoverished or rural patients. Patients without reliable, private transportation cannot easily access some services, even if available and affordable.

♦ *Probability of payer approval.* Even if the optimal treatment plan is available, whether the insurance carrier or other third-party payer will approve it remains an open question. Anyone who has struggled to convince a health maintenance organization (HMO) to approve an extended hospital or residential treatment knows of what we speak.

♦ *Caregiver approval.* The research and the practitioner may agree on an optimal treatment plan, but the parents or caregiver may not. For children and adolescents, the referring caregivers, rather than the identified patient, will likely choose the therapist and make other treatment decisions. However, children naturally have their own preferences and agendas.

♦ *Incongruous recommendations.* At the national level, different behavioral health disciplines offer disparate, even competing treatment guidelines. At the local level, professionals from different disciplines may offer disparate treatment plans. For example, a cocaine addict who recently consulted us was offered, in the course of several weeks, four different "evidence based" treatments. A psychologist recommended intensive outpatient psychotherapy (without medication), a psychiatrist recommended outpatient medication (without psychotherapy), an addictions counselor recommended inpatient detoxification and 14-day rehabilitation, and a pastoral counselor recommended Cocaine Anonymous and spiritual counseling.

♦ *Prior treatment failures.* Many patients present with chronic histories both of their long-term suffering and of many unsuccessful treatment episodes, including with EBPs. "Been there, done that" is a familiar refrain among patients in community clinics.

♦ *Intolerable side effects.* Some patients cannot tolerate the side effects of the finest research-supported treatments, whether psychotropic medications or intense psychotherapies.

Take the case of Francesco. He has no insurance coverage and little money. Even if he could obtain a few free or low-cost sessions of outpatient therapy for his generalized anxiety disorder (GAD) from his case manager, he would probably not receive a cutting-edge, state-of-the-art EBP treatment. In all likelihood, Francesco would receive a prescription for an antianxiety medication from his

primary-care physician. His enrolling in an extensive alcohol rehabilitation program seems improbable given his lack of health insurance and inability to pay privately. And even if that possibility were
offered, Francesco's low readiness to change would probably lead him
to decline at this time. Moreover, Francesco's chronic history of alcohol dependence, two previous inpatient rehabilitations, and current
minimization of his substance abuse all conspire to lower his odds of
a good prognosis without extensive treatment.

Any EBP that does not consider the patient's unique characteristics, culture, and preferences is ripe for failure. This necessary
element of EBP entails shared decision-making and ongoing consultation with patients. Fortunately, mental health professionals
(and their ethical codes) prize patient autonomy and empowerment.
Eliciting treatment priorities, establishing consensus on treatment
goals, ascertaining client cultures of import, sharing the pros and
cons of alternatives, considering socioeconomic resources, collaborating on the way forward, and continually monitoring progress
toward the goals all represent fundamental skills of behavioral health
practitioners.

Decision aids can help patients make informed decisions
about the best health treatments among multiple alternatives.
Such aids can also prove useful when no option has a clear advantage in terms of outcome and when each option has benefits and
harms that patients value differently. Videos, pamphlets, Web-
based materials, and other aids can make the decision explicit,
describe the available alternatives, and explicate the possible benefits and risks. A Cochrane Review of 115 studies, encompassing
more than 34,000 patients, found that patients who employed
decision aids improved their knowledge of the options, felt more
informed about what mattered most to them, held more accurate
expectations of possible benefits and harms, and participated more
actively in final decisions compared with patients who did not use
such aids (Stacey et al., 2014). Indeed, decision aids improve communication between practitioners and patients. The research and
practice in this area to date have been conducted overwhelmingly
on biophysical treatments; in the EBP tradition, we fully expect
decision aids to become more frequently used in behavioral health
and addiction practice.

Skill Exercise 9-1

Practice and perhaps role-play shared decision-making with potential patients about treatment selections. Rehearse how you will introduce the subject and how you will present the key considerations (e.g., demonstrated efficacy, potential harms, underlying values, patient fit, prior treatment experiences, and payer approval). Here are several scenarios involving choices among research-supported treatments: interpersonal therapy versus cognitive–behavioral therapy for bulimia; psychotherapy versus exercise versus antidepressant medication for depression; individual therapy versus group therapy for social anxiety; individual therapy versus parent management training for a child with ADHD; abstinence-based versus harm reduction therapies for problem drinking; and individual versus family therapy for adolescent drug abuse. Avoid the tendency to present "both" as an option, since practical, temporal, and economic restraints frequently preclude the ideal combination.

Clinicians can commit the error of underestimating the uniqueness of patients, on the one hand, or overstating the uniqueness of patients, on the other. Having now emphasized the former, let us remind ourselves of the folly of the latter. If we place undue, exaggerated emphasis on patient uniqueness, we may undercut the potential influence of clinical research findings. We may then fall prey to the heuristic (see Chapter 10) of justifying what we are accustomed to doing regardless of the research evidence (G. T. Wilson, 1995). Proper EBP entails thoughtfully and impartially integrating all three components.

Integrating the Three Components

The EBP trinity—best research, clinical expertise, and patient characteristics, cultures, and preferences—is not an equal partnership. Research stands as the first and primary source of evidence.

According to our (and others') definition, EBP practitioners integrate research with clinical expertise in the context of patient characteristics, culture, and preferences.

Evidence-based practice decisions occur at the intersection of these three components, as graphically illustrated in Figure 9.1 (based on Walker et al., 2006). This Venn diagram portrays an ideal situation in which the research literature, clinical expertise, and patient characteristics largely converge. The substantial overlap indicates that all three evidentiary sources are largely in agreement on how to proceed in practice—whether in assessment, prevention, or treatment. If only all decisions proved so consensual and easy!

Consider the assessment and treatment of Annique's recurrent major depression. Research tells us that several psychometrically sound and clinically useful measures can assess her depression and monitor her symptom improvement (or deterioration) throughout the course of treatment. As a bright and informed patient, Annique concurs that periodic assessment of her depression would serve her well. Such assessment fits congruently with her preferences and values. Her private-practice psychologist knows the research on the assessment of depression and routinely employs self-report depression measures every third or fifth session. Similarly, the research evidence, the clinician's expertise, and Annique's preferences all align with interpersonal psychotherapy (IPT), an evidence-based

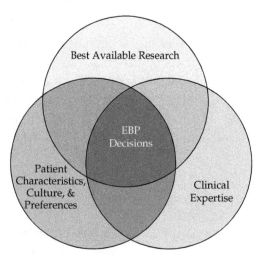

FIGURE 9.1 Venn diagram illustrating substantial convergence among all three EBP components.

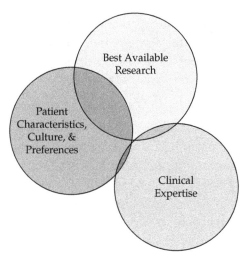

FIGURE 9.2 Venn diagram illustrating substantial convergence between available research and patient preferences but minimal overlap with clinical expertise.

psychotherapy for treatment of acute depression and prevention of its recurrence. The research, clinical expertise, and patient values all converge—an optimal, Figure 9.1-type situation.

Figure 9.2 displays a clinical case in which the patient values and research evidence overlap but the practitioner's expertise remains out of sync with both. Two of the circles overlap considerably with each other but not with the third circle. Here, the clinical decision is decidedly more complex and challenging.

To continue with our example, suppose that Annique and the research both support IPT (or another research-supported treatment, say, cognitive–behavioral therapy, short-term psychodynamic therapy, or emotion-focused therapy). However, the practitioner favors Therapy X, which Annique does not prefer and for which no controlled outcome research exists for acute or maintenance treatment of depression. The practitioner has skill in rendering diagnoses, conceptualizing cases, forming facilitative relationships, and other critical areas but lacks both training in IPT and the inclination to obtain it (or, for the sake of illustration, the other research-supported therapies for major depression).

How to proceed toward a clinical decision? In the face of evidence that IPT works for this disorder, it is not sufficient for the practitioner who prefers Therapy X to rest on the fact that no one has proven it ineffective. The research-supported treatment remains the EBP and probably the most ethical choice in the majority of cases.

Nonetheless, in some cases, other factors will mitigate that consideration. Three such mitigating factors are:

♦ Recently available controlled research documents the success of Therapy X.
♦ In the process of obtaining informed consent, the clinician describes the alternatives and the evidence for each, permitting the client to make an educated decision in favor of Therapy X. (Recognize, however, that a depressed and dependent patient like Annique might well uncritically accede to a clinician's theoretical inclinations if strongly expressed.)
♦ Annique has undergone treatment on two occasions with the research-supported psychotherapy but has not improved, and now the clinician persuades her that they should opt for an alternative treatment.

Absent such mitigating circumstances, the ethics codes of behavioral health professions argue in favor of offering research-supported treatments. The clinician need not have proficiency in all treatments and may thus refer Annique elsewhere if he is not trained in the EBP. We believe that most clinicians would, in fact, refer Annique to a colleague offering the indicated treatment should she maintain her strong treatment preference for the EBP.

Another clinical situation frequently occurs as well: The practitioner's expertise and the best research overlap, but they diverge from the patient's preferences and culture. Figure 9.3 depicts this clinical situation.

In Annique's case, this scenario would occur when the best available research and clinical expertise converge in recommending the EBPs of IPT (or another research-supported therapies) and antidepressant medication to treat her recurrent depression, but she rejects these. Annique might

♦ elect to discontinue antidepressant medications because of intolerable side effects or a philosophical objection to "chemical solutions";
♦ prefer a psychotherapy specifically developed for and evaluated on African American women;

- ◆ opt for a discredited treatment, say, sitting an hour a day in an orgone energy accumulator to absorb (nonexistent) orgone energy (Norcross et al., 2006b); or
- ◆ decide that her primary goal in this course of psychotherapy lies in developing insight into the intrapsychic and family origins of her depression, as opposed to focusing on symptom reduction. In such a case, an EBP primarily devoted to and validated in research on symptom reduction might not be the treatment of choice. More than 90% of outcome measures in published behavioral health RCTs concern symptoms (Farnsworth et al., 2001).

Jonathon's case provides an exemplar of the clinical situation portrayed in Figure 9.3. The research supports the efficacy of parent management training, stimulant medication, and classroom management for Jonathon's ADHD. The clinical expertise of the practitioner supports all three treatments. Yet Jonathon's father firmly resists any psychotropic medication, taking that EBP off the table, at least in the short run. Both parents express a willingness to participate in a few family meetings, but their demanding work schedules and marital conflicts prevent extensive outpatient treatment. Can parent management training deliver its benefits in a few sessions with discordant parents? Perhaps Jonathon's elementary school runs a

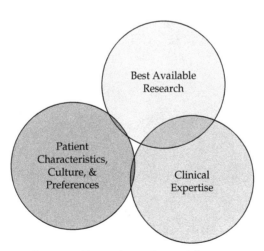

FIGURE 9.3 Venn diagram illustrating substantial convergence between available research and clinical expertise but minimal overlap with patient preferences and culture.

classroom behavior management program, but the teacher already feels overwhelmed by the needs of the other 29 children in her classroom and insists that the parents medicate Jonathon. She advocates for special services for Jonathon in the classroom; if these are not provided, she argues for his being placed in a substantially separate classroom for the emotionally disturbed.

Figure 9.4 illustrates yet another decision-making scenario: The patient's values and the clinician's expertise align well, but the best research stands apart. Annique, to continue with our example, presents to psychotherapy with definite culturally driven preferences for an African American female therapist who will actively engage Annique's larger community, including her church group and pastor, in her psychological treatment. Meta-analyses show that ethnic minority clients definitely prefer ethnically similar therapists over European American therapists (Cabral & Smith, 2011) but that ethnic minority therapists achieve no better or worse treatment outcomes (Cabral & Smith, 2011; Sue & Lam, 2002). Hundreds of controlled research studies have investigated the efficacy of family and community interventions, but none, based on our knowledge and literature search, specifically involved church groups in the treatment of depression. So Annique's preferences enjoy no support in the controlled

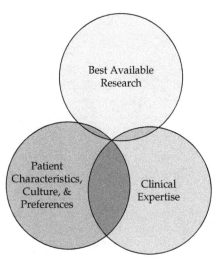

FIGURE 9.4 Venn diagram illustrating substantial convergence between clinical expertise and patient preferences and culture but minimal overlap with available research.

research, but neither do we find data in the research literature to contradict them. Annique's preferred therapist, an African American woman, possesses training and competence in working with larger systems, views therapy as a collaborative endeavor, and responds effectively to patients' values and preferences. She works with Annique's inclinations to their mutual satisfaction. Although this particular treatment approach would not appear on a list of "evidence based" treatments or in a practice guideline, their treatment plan certainly qualifies as "evidence based" in the best sense of that term.

Another situation in which patient characteristics and clinical expertise trump the research-supported treatment is when the values of the patient contrast with those embodied within the research-supported intervention. Annique might decide that restructuring her relationships in IPT or her cognitions in cognitive therapy does not coincide with her worldview. She elects a spiritual or existential psychotherapy whose philosophy feels more congruent with her personal values. Clinical expertise would lead most professionals to determine that such therapy probably holds the greatest probability of benefit, given the strength of Annique's values and the possible iatrogenic effect of imposing a treatment against those values. One goal of EBP is to maximize patient choice among effective alternative interventions (APA Task Force on Evidence-Based Practice, 2006).

In the interest of completeness, we should acknowledge one final, logical relationship among the three EBP components: All three spheres barely overlap with one another. We have found this to occur very rarely in ordinary practice. Almost always, at least two of the components overlap considerably.

Complex Cases

What works in behavioral health and addiction treatment? The definitive answer, the only evidence-based answer, is "It depends." Successful intervention necessarily considers the individuality of the patient, the singularity of the context, the nature of the patient's problems, the availability of resources, the likely prognosis, and the expected benefits. Frequently, in the words of Sir William Osler (1906), the father of modern medicine, "It is much more important to know what sort of a patient has a disease than what sort of disease a patient has."

Many of our cases are, in a word, complex. In fact, practitioners' concerns about the value of EBPs for complex patients, who may differ in significant ways from the samples in clinical trials, contribute to the underutilization of EBP (Ruscio & Holohan, 2006). Patient complexity can manifest in many ways, as summarized in Box 9.1. All types of patient complexity tend to decrease a favorable prognosis, and all complicate the integration of best research with clinical expertise and patient contributions. But ironically, it is exactly with complex and perplexing cases that practitioners most often seek evidence-based guidance.

It would prove impossible to discuss all the features of complex cases listed in Box 9.1 in a brief, how-to manual on EBPs. Nonetheless, we can profitably work a couple of examples to demonstrate the process of arriving at an EBP decision with a complex case.

Consider the clinical complexity of working with intellectually disabled clients, who statistically represent 1% of the population but 5–10% of the behavioral health population. Can prevention and treatment RCTs conducted on the intellectually abled generalize to the other 1%? Or should we confine ourselves to the impressive but largely uncontrolled intervention research performed with intellectually disabled adults?

 Skill Exercise 9-2

A well-tested set of therapeutic strategies have proved highly effective for depression and anxiety, but all of the RCTs published have excluded individuals with IQ/index scores below 80 and with thought disorders. You work in a practice setting that frequently serves depressed and anxious adults with below-average IQs and those in recovery from schizophrenia. Describe how you might go about making appropriate use of the extant research with your patients.

Comorbid disorders confound any simple or linear determination of a treatment plan from the research evidence. Ponder the frequent co-occurrence of major depression and GAD. In a prospective longitudinal study, a birth **cohort** of 1,037 people was

Box 9.1 Common Features of Complex Cases

Symptom presentations

> Severe symptoms
> Chronic course
> Comorbid disorders
> Severe functional impairment in multiple domains
> Symptoms maintained by factors that are difficult to change
> Presenting problem generally considered difficult to treat
> No EBPs available for presenting disorders

Legal entanglements

> Court-mandated treatment
> Secondary gain to preserve impairment, e.g., in disability
>   evaluations
> Strong motivation to present or fake "good," e.g., in child
>   custody evaluations
> Repeated charges or formal complaints against healthcare
>   professionals

Suicide and safety concerns

> Suicidal and self-destructive behaviors
> Parasuicidal or self-injurious behaviors
> Past suicide attempts
> Homicidal impulses or tendencies
> Frequent hospitalizations
> Ongoing physical danger

Physical/medical complications

> Chronic pain
> Multiple, diffuse somatic symptoms
> Medical condition causing psychological symptoms
> Physical disability maintaining psychological condition
> Physical factors limiting treatment

Intellectual limitations

Limited intellectual ability
Low education level
Cognitive impairment

Interpersonal impediments

Personality disorders that undermine the therapeutic alliance
Severe personality traits, e.g., hostility, suspiciousness, dependence
Pervasive tendency to externalize problems
Low psychological mindedness
Low self-esteem or self-efficacy

Psychosocial factors

History of chronic or repeated trauma
Multiple, significant stressors
Severe financial instability
Social isolation
Unstable or insecure social environment
Family and social system undermining treatment

Motivational factors

Severe hopelessness and demoralization
Precontemplation stage (denial of problems)
High level of reactance/resistance
Low expectancy for improvement
Strong commitment to problematic beliefs or behaviors
External contingencies reinforcing the sick role
Poor commitment to therapy
Treatment noncompliance

Treatment history

Repeated prior treatment failures
History of premature termination and dropout
Unsuccessful prior treatment with EBPs

Adapted from Ruscio & Holohan (2006).

followed to age 32 years (with an impressive retention of 96%). Cumulatively, 72% of lifetime anxiety cases from this group demonstrated a history of depression, and 48% of lifetime depression cases also had anxiety. In this comorbid group, depression onset occurred first in one third of the participants, anxiety onset occurred first in one third of the participants, and depression and anxiety onset began concurrently in the remaining third of the cases (Moffitt et al., 2007).

Presenting with major depression, Annique has almost a 50% chance of experiencing clinical levels of anxiety as well. Presenting with GAD, Francesco has a 72% chance of experiencing clinical depression at some point. As every seasoned psychotherapist knows, anxiety and depression rarely present as discrete disorders.

> The book's companion website contains hyperlinks to a dozen recommended websites on comorbid/co-occurring mental health disorders and dual diagnoses.

The cultural context challenges us to think in terms of idiographic cases as contrasted to the normative probabilities of group research. Does the applicability of research results depend, for example, on the nation and time period? Case in point: Does your view of the applicability of the research evidence from the prospective longitudinal study mentioned above change when you learn that the study took place in Dunedin, New Zealand, starting in 1972–1973? To what extent should we base the probability of comorbid diagnoses for Annique and Francesco on such findings?

The chronicity and ego-dystonic nature of personality disorders add layers of complexity to clinical decisions. Treating patients suffering from personality disorders is notoriously challenging because of the difficulties they experience in building a reliable therapeutic alliance and cooperating in corrective actions. The prevalence of personality disorders proves high across most mental disorders; for example, 37% of drug addicts and 53% of alcohol abusers simultaneously suffer from at least one personality disorder (Bowden-Jones et al., 2004). Moreover, diagnoses of individuals with two or more personality disorders are astonishingly frequent; based on the criteria from the fourth edition of the *Diagnostic and Statistical Manual of Mental Disorders* (DSM-IV; APA, 1994), patients with schizotypal personality disorder have an average of 2.4 additional personality disorders, and patients with borderline personality disorder have 1.9 more concurrent personality disorders (McGlashan et al., 2000).

 Skill Exercise 9-3

Investigate the availability of meta-analyses and systematic reviews of RCTs in the treatment of comorbid mental disorders as well as of concurrent personality disorders. Select a couple of filtered information sources from among those discussed in Chapter 3 (e.g., the Cochrane Database, NREPP, and discipline-specific websites) and determine whether you can find a useful summary of the research literature. Could you readily locate such research reviews on the treatment of comorbid mental disorders and personality disorders? (Nor could we, at least as of spring 2016.)

Then we have that subset of patients who present with high levels of reactance or resistance, meaning that they become easily provoked and respond oppositionally to external demands. High client resistance is associated with poorer therapy outcomes in 82% of studies. Fortunately, research (Beutler et al., 2011b) has determined that matching therapist directiveness to client level of resistance improved therapy outcome in 16 of 20 studies (80%). Specifically, clients presenting with high resistance benefit more from self-control methods, minimal therapist directiveness, and **paradoxical interventions**. By contrast, clients with low resistance benefit more from therapist directiveness and explicit guidance.

Note that these research conclusions come from multiple studies conducted across patient diagnoses. That is, they represent **transdiagnostic** patterns. Such studies stand in contrast to the overwhelming majority of RCTs on treatment efficacy, which include patients from a single diagnostic category.

In order to sensitively integrate the research with the patient and the clinician, we increasingly need to know not simply which treatments work for which disorder but which treatments work for which person. Different folks demand different strokes. Here, it seems to us, lies the central difference between EBPs in medicine and EBPs in behavioral health: the relentless complexity of people. We do not minimize the complexity of the physical body or disease states. Rather, behavioral health and addiction professionals address all of that pathology complexity on top of the immense complexity of human behavior.

Adopt, Adapt, or Abandon

After evaluating the confluence of the three components of EBP and considering the complexity of patient characteristics, we must make a clinical decision and act accordingly. Practitioners have three basic options for a particular patient with regard to a research-supported intervention: **Adopt it, adapt it, or abandon it**. Given the seemingly infinite number of competing considerations, the evidence-based practitioner confronts difficult decisions in many cases.

We *adopt* the research-supported EBP when we believe it qualifies as a "good enough" fit for the particular patient and context. Providing the EBP in its original form affords several benefits (Ruscio & Holohan, 2006):

◆ The treatment has been tested and has been demonstrated as efficacious for alleviating the target problem, thus maximizing the probability of client success.
◆ The clinician will probably feel more confident in using an EBP and will communicate that confidence to the patient.
◆ The client, as a part of informed consent, will learn that she is receiving a demonstrably effective, scientifically supported treatment with low attrition.

In our experience, the majority of behavioral health and addiction patients make a good enough match with at least one EBP for one or more of their presenting problems.

We *adapt* an EBP when we believe it has utility but does not quite seem adequate for the particular patient, problem, and context. Adaptations can entail modifying, supplementing, or sequencing the treatment in ways not studied in the research trials in order to accommodate the needs of the patient. The obvious advantages of adaptation include the belief that the treatment aligns better with the patient's needs and that the proven efficacy of the EBP will generalize to this case. The disadvantages include the unknown impact of the adaptation on the efficacy of treatment and the possibility that the modified EBP loses its curative ingredients. Indeed, early research suggests that adapting research-supported treatments for specific disorders to an individual patient seldom improves treatment outcome (Ruscio & Holohan, 2006). However, adapting EBPs may mean the difference between making some treatment gains by engaging the patient and making no treatment gains at all by imposing a treatment the patient deems unacceptable.

Resolving the conflict between **fidelity** and fit, both essential elements of EBP, creates dynamic tension. We seek fidelity of implementation in the delivery of the manualized intervention found effective in controlled research. At the same time, we seek fit in adapting the service to the needs of the specific patient (Castro et al., 2004).

A series of meta-analytic reviews compiled by an APA intradivisional task force (Norcross, 2011) identified research-supported ways to adapt psychological therapies to six transdiagnostic features of patients: reactance level, stages of change, preferences, coping style, religion or spirituality, and culture. Think of these as "when . . . then" principles: When clients present with certain characteristics, then the research evidence supports an adaptation. These principles represent person–treatment, not disorder–treatment, matches. We discussed adaptation to high reactance levels above; the following are thumbnail descriptions of adaptations for the other five transdiagnostic features:

◆ *Stages of change.* The amount of progress clients make in psychotherapy tends to be a direct function of their pretreatment stage of change—precontemplation, contemplation, preparation, action, and maintenance. A meta-analysis of 39 psychotherapy studies (Norcross et al., 2011) found a mean effect size d of 0.46, indicating that the stages reliably predict outcomes. More importantly, a meta-analysis (Rosen, 2000) of 47 research studies demonstrated that different processes of change are differentially effective in certain stages of change ($d = 0.70$ and 0.80). That is, adapting psychotherapy to the client's stage of change significantly improves outcome across disorders (Prochaska & Norcross, 2014). Action-oriented therapies are quite effective with individuals who are in the preparation or action stages. However, these same therapies tend to be less effective or even detrimental with individuals in the precontemplation and contemplation stages.

◆ *Preferences.* The patient's preferences and goals are frequently direct indicators of the best therapeutic method and healing relationship for that person. Decades of empirical evidence attest to the benefit of seriously considering, and at least beginning psychotherapy in accordance with, the relational preferences and treatment goals of the client. A meta-analysis of 35 studies compared the treatment outcomes of clients matched to their preferred treatments to outcomes of those clients not matched to their preferences. The findings indicated a medium positive effect ($d = 0.31$) in favor of clients matched to preferences. Clients who were matched to their preferences were one third less likely to drop out of psychotherapy—a powerful effect indeed (Swift et al., 2011).

◆ *Coping style.* The research on coping styles has been devoted primarily to the externalizing (impulsive, stimulation seeking, extroverted) and internalizing (self-critical, inhibited, introverted) styles. A meta-analysis of 12 studies involving more than a thousand patients revealed a medium effect ($d = 0.55$) for matching therapist method to patient coping style (Beutler et al., 2011a). Specifically, interpersonal and insight-oriented therapies are more effective among internalizing patients, whereas symptom-focused and skill-building therapies are more effective among externalizing patients. This person–treatment fit is familiar to clinicians for child patients—in treating, say, a depressed internalizing girl versus a hyperactive externalizing boy—but less well known for the adult patients on whom the meta-analysis was conducted.

◆ *Religion/spirituality.* In 29 studies with 3,290 patients, those receiving religiously or spiritually adapted therapies showed greater improvement than those in alternative, secular psychotherapies on both psychological ($d = 0.26$) and spiritual ($d = 0.41$) outcomes. However, in 11 more rigorous dismantling designs, in which religious/spiritual and alternative treatments shared the same theoretical orientation and treatment duration, no differences in psychological outcomes were noted, though differences in spiritual outcomes ($d = 0.33$) favored the religiously or spiritually accommodative therapies (Worthington et al., 2011). In other words, using a religiously or spiritually adapted therapy when requested by a patient provided equivalent treatment outcomes on psychological measures and better spiritual outcomes.

Skill Exercise 9-4

A client has sought your services for help in overcoming social anxiety, but balks when you propose a well-researched intervention supported by numerous RCTs. The client cites religious values that proscribe some of the methods you describe as components of the manualized treatment. How would you respond to this objection? (Hint: Consider the three options of adopting it, adapting it, or abandoning it; as well, consider the cost–benefit ratio of convincing the patient to accept your proposed treatment and requesting the involvement of the patient's clergy to respond to the client's objections.)

◆ *Culture.* A meta-analysis of 65 studies encompassing 8,620 clients evaluated the effectiveness of culturally adapted therapies versus traditional, nonadapted therapies. The most frequent methods of adaptation in the studies involved incorporating cultural content and values, using the client's preferred language, and matching clients to therapists of similar ethnicity. The results revealed a positive effect ($d = 0.46$) in favor of clients' receiving culturally adapted treatments (T. B. Smith et al., 2011). Cultural "fit" works, not only as an ethical commitment but also as an EBP.

Consider two examples of **cultural adaptation** of research-supported interventions—one in substance abuse prevention and the other in parent management training. An innovative substance abuse prevention program in the Southwest built in a cultural adaptation to enhance program fit while maintaining fidelity of implementation (Castro et al., 2004). The adaptation involved modifying some program content and the form of program delivery. The latter included characteristics of the clinicians (lay health workers rather than health educators), the channel by which services were delivered (on the Internet rather than in formal presentations), and the location of services (a community hall rather than a school classroom).

Parent management training has a long and well-established evidence base (Kazdin, 2005) but has shown some racial and ethnic disparities in outcomes (Lau, 2006). The wide variation in parenting practices and family values across ethnic groups has led many researchers to adapt the treatment. Some changes lie at the surface, such as including community-relevant examples, modifying pictures to depict ethnically similar families, and respecting cultural values. Other changes are more structural—for example, recruiting in community networks, matching the ethnicity of the clinician to the clientele, conducting the treatment groups in churches, and addressing basic living needs. The outcomes of the adapted parent training typically equate to outcomes for the standard versions; however, the cultural adaptation frequently results in marked improvements in client recruitment, satisfaction, and retention (Lau, 2006).

Of course, adaptation of EBPs to cultural contexts and other patient characteristics must be systematically guided by research evidence. Research can identify target problems and communities that would most benefit from an adaptation and then direct the design of the treatment adaptation (Lau, 2006). We also need to factor in the bottom-line question of whether the outcomes justify the additional costs of cultural adaptation. The consensus in the field points to routinely making adaptations for person–treatment (transdiagnostic) matches but being more selective about disorder–treatment (diagnostic) adaptations.

We *abandon* a research-supported intervention either before treatment commences, because we believe it does not apply to the particular patient and context, or during treatment when it does not produce the desired results. Before treatment, clinicians may decide that the research-supported intervention lacks applicability and generalizability (for one or more of the reasons reviewed in Chapter 8 and in this chapter). During treatment, clinicians may decide to abandon the research-supported option because the patient shows signs of deteriorating, is not making progress, refuses to continue, threatens to drop out, or insists on an alternative.

When treatment with a research-supported intervention is failing, the clinician can proceed in many ways. Possible strategies include

- determining, in a nonblaming style with the patient, the reasons that the current treatment is not working;
- revisiting the therapeutic contract and asking if the treatment had a sufficient chance, or "dose," to work;
- adapting the research-supported treatment in some manner;
- delaying or resequencing the treatment;
- returning to the literature to discover other research-supported practices for the particular patient and context;

♦ reconsidering the patient's diagnoses and treatment goals;
♦ evaluating the patient's readiness to change or motivational level;
♦ evaluating the therapeutic relationship, particularly for ruptures in the therapeutic alliance;
♦ obtaining peer consultation or supervision on the case; and
♦ transferring the patient to another clinician.

The Reflective, Evidence-Based Practitioner

Decision trees (see Figures 8.1 and 8.2), Venn diagrams (Figures 9.1–9.4), and case examples can only begin to capture the enormous complexity of integrating the best available research with clinical expertise and patient characteristics, cultures, and preferences. Risk–benefit analyses, likelihood ratios, and decisional balances are humble paths through the tangled thicket of complex and conflicting considerations. Sensitive application and thoughtful integration of the research can be taxing. At times, we secretly crave the older, discarded practice of mindlessly providing all patients with the identical treatment!

But clinical experience and controlled research convincingly demonstrate the error of that old way. Michels (1984, p. xiii) has written:

> The easiest way to practice is to view all patients and problems as basically the same, and to apply one standard therapy for their treatment. Although some may still employ this model, everything we have learned in recent decades tells us that it is wrong—wrong for our patients in that it deprives them of the most effective treatment, and wrong for everyone else in that it wastes scarce resources.

His words underscore the overarching purposes of EBP, which, as you will recall from Chapter 1, are to improve the care of the individual patient and to enhance the health of the entire population.

In the end, the practitioner performs the integration with skill, flexibility, scientific attitude, and cultural sensitivity while monitoring patient progress and adjusting treatment as necessary. We rely on research but soberly acknowledge that not all research applies to our current situation and that individual patients may require decisions and interventions not directly addressed by the available research. Effective practice requires delicate balancing, recursive decision-making, and collaborative relationships to ensure that patients understand the probable costs, risks, and benefits of different choices.

Key Terms

adopt it, adapt it, or abandon it
clinical expertise
cohort
comorbid disorders
cultural adaptation
decision aids

fidelity
paradoxical interventions
patient characteristics, culture,
    and preferences
transdiagnostic

Recommended Readings and Websites

Bohart, A. C., & Tallman, K. (1999). *How clients make therapy work: The process of active self-healing.* Washington, DC: American Psychological Association.

Bernal, G., & Domenech Rodriguez, M. M. (Eds.). (2012). *Cultural adaptations: Tools for evidence-based practice with diverse populations.* Washington, DC: American Psychological Association.

Centre for Evidence-Based Medicine. Applying Evidence to Patients, ktclearinghouse.ca/cebm/practise/apply

DiClemente, C. C. (2006). *Addiction and change: How addictions develop and addicted people recover.* New York, NY: Guilford.

Hunink, M. G. M., Weinstein, M. C., Wittenberg, E., Drummond, M. F., Pliskin, J. S., Wong, J. B., & Glasziou, P. P. (2014). *Decision making in health and medicine: Integrating evidence and values* (2nd ed.). Cambridge, UK: Cambridge University Press.

Lambert, M. J. (Ed.). (2013). *Bergin and Garfield's handbook of psychotherapy and behavior change* (6th ed.). New York, NY: Wiley.

Norcross, J. C. (Ed.). (2011). *Psychotherapy relationships that work* (2nd ed.). New York, NY: Oxford University Press.

10

Incorporating Evaluation
and Ethics

The final core step in evidence-based practice (EBP) involves evaluating the effectiveness of the entire process. That's the final *E*(valuation) in AAA TIE. In the literature, this skill is typically referred to as monitoring, measuring, or auditing clinical performance. In this chapter we look at clinical performance at three levels of evaluation: the individual practitioner, the program or administrative unit, and the profession as a whole. We also address readiness for change and how to carry an ethical focus forward in caring for our patients, evaluating ourselves, and managing risk.

We can track the evaluation process using the stages of change often used to describe behavior change and psychotherapy progress (Norcross, 2013; Prochaska et al., 1995). Individual practitioners will move through five stages—precontemplation, contemplation, preparation, action, and maintenance—as they adapt their work and implement EBP.

By taking this book seriously you have demonstrated movement past precontemplation and probably even past contemplation. You have gone beyond the "Who cares about EBP?" attitude of the precontemplator and probably past the "Do I really want to do this?"

of the contemplator. You have plunged in deeply and should feel prepared to take action. This will likely require altering your practice in significant ways and may necessitate continuing education to acquire familiarity with new assessment, prevention, or treatment approaches. Success will also require follow-through and follow-up (i.e., implementing the EBPs and evaluating the outcome of your work). Table 10.1 enumerates the stages of change as applied to EBP in behavioral health and addictions.

This chapter begins with an evaluation of EBP implementation at three levels: the individual practitioner, the program or administrative unit, and the profession as a whole. We then

TABLE 10.1 Stages of Change in Adoption of Evidence-Based Practice (EBP)

Stage of change relative to EBP	Characteristic questioning	Suggestions for promoting movement
Precontemplation	Who cares about EBP? The status quo is fine with me.	Encourage re-evaluation and self-exploration; recognize risks of doing nothing.
Contemplation	Do I really want to do this? What are the benefits and risks?	Consider the pros and cons of adopting EBPs, including potential positive outcomes.
Preparation	Okay, I bought the book and am intrigued. Now what?	Identify any obstacles, acquire necessary skills, and begin taking small steps.
Action	I want to do it, but can I? Let's see how this goes.	Practice the core EBP skills, improve self-efficacy, and focus on long-term benefits.
Maintenance	Can I sustain this? How did I ever do without it?	Follow up and document patients' successes, prevent relapse, and promote self-reinforcement.

focus on risk management, liability standards, and ethical issues—matters typically and tragically too often ignored when considering EBPs.

Evaluating One's Own Performance

A good evaluation of an individual practitioner's performance involves both self-evaluation and evaluation by others. One might think that well-intentioned, highly educated, clinically skilled practitioners trained in EBP would know about their own skill level based on introspective self-awareness. However, quoting from the lyrics of George Gershwin in *Porgy and Bess*, "It ain't necessarily so." Difficulties in recognizing one's own incompetence can easily lead people to hold overly favorable views of their abilities in many contexts (Kruger & Dunning, 1999). Personal biases and the intense wish for one's patients to improve further complicate objective assessment of outcomes in mental health and the addictions.

Humans absorb and process massive amounts of sensory data and attempt to make sense of it all using organizing strategies or cognitive anchors. But these usually are not probabilistic cognitive processes; sadly, most humans think nonprobabilistically. We typically attempt to insert new data into our preexisting worldviews as opposed to expanding our thinking outward based on the new data or observations. Some people refer to these human organizing strategies as **heuristics**—"mental rules of thumb" that we use to perform abstract reasoning in cognitively economical ways. These strategies generally operate below our threshold of awareness and save us time and effort, but they often fail when we are confronted by data at variance with or outside of our domains of expertise.

Such failures often tend to pass without notice. For one thing, the cognitive processes responsible for judging the quality of our thinking fall prey to these biases as well. For another, these biases apply so broadly and seem so natural that few people notice them. Finally, decisions made based on heuristics often simply feel good or correct. Such ways of conceptualizing our world leave us intuitively satisfied regardless of their correctness. Table 10.2 lists some important heuristic biases.

TABLE 10.2 Examples of Heuristic Biases

Name	Description
Anchoring effect	Failure to make sufficient adjustments away from initial anchor points, even when the points are arbitrary
Availability bias	Preferential use of ideas that come to mind more easily, typically associated with high imagery (e.g., people's estimates of the likelihood or frequency of being struck by lightning or winning the lottery, uninformed by actual odds)
Base rate neglect	Overlooking background frequencies in favor of anecdotal evidence (e.g., "All my clients are liberal Democrats, so . . .")
Confirmation bias	Seeking out opinions and facts that support our own beliefs and hypotheses (e.g., "I'm sure I'm right, I just need to find the proof")
Conjunction fallacy	A logical contradiction in which the joint probability of two events (e.g., that Jonathon both gets good grades and likes baseball) is seen as higher than the independent probabilities of each—a literal mathematical impossibility
False consensus bias	Inclination to assume your beliefs are more widely held than they actually are (e.g., "Family therapists pretty much agree on this")
Fortune teller effect (or Barnum effect)	Tendency of people to accept general descriptions as uniquely relevant to them (e.g., "You think about sex from time to time")
Framing effect	Disparities in estimates when identical problems or data are arrayed in different configurations or sequences
Gambler's fallacy	Pervasive false beliefs about the nature of random sequences (e.g., "I've lost so many times that I'm due for a win any time now")

TABLE 10.2 Continued

Name	Description
Groupthink	Pressure to irrationally agree with others in strong team-based cultures (e.g., "I better keep my odd ideas to myself because the rest of the team thinks the sky is green")
Homogeneity bias	Exaggerated conclusions about large populations based on small samples (e.g., "My three clients typify the universe")
Lake Wobegon effect	Tendency for all people to assume they are above average (named after folk humorist Garrison Keillor's fictional town)
Misperceptions of randomness	Systematic errors in judging the randomness of events (e.g., rating a seemingly patterned sequence of heads [H] or tails [T] coin tosses, such as HHHTTT, as less likely than a less patterned sequence, such as HTHTTH, even though the sequences have exactly the same probability of occurring)
"Not my fault" bias	Tendency to attribute failures to other people (e.g., "If my patient didn't improve, she must have not followed my advice or screwed up some other way")
Representativeness bias	Drawing inferences by using a prototype to represent a category, while ignoring base rates (e.g., assuming that a person is a criminal or has committed a criminal act because he has similarities to a general notion of criminals)
Truthiness	Coined by comedian Stephen Colbert, the human propensity for determining truth by what we feel in our gut, independent of and frequently in opposition to objective reality or scientific research
Wow effect	Letting emotional memories override normative reasoning

Skill Exercise 10-1

Review Table 10.2 and then (a) identify those heuristic biases that probably operate in your own thinking about clinical matters and (b) invent your own heuristic bias. Do so by identifying some common approach to conceptualizing or categorizing people or events in a way that leads to faulty judgments.

How might various heuristics play out in the clinical context? *Confirmation bias* may lead the clinician to see success where expected and to overlook evidence of failure. When clinicians tap their memories for a treatment method that worked with similar clients in the past, they risk making decisions biased on the *wow effect* or *homogeneity bias*: Thinking of examples of an intervention's particularly memorable success or failure will influence estimations of the likelihood that the treatment will help in the present case; one or two successful cases may prove sufficient to override the memory of cases for which the same approach did not work. The *"not my fault" bias* comes into play when clinicians' self-assessments lead them to ascribe treatment failures to clients' behaviors or characteristics while attributing successes in treatment to themselves and their skills.

What does the research evidence tell us about countering such heuristics? The strategy of simply informing people about a particular bias and warning them to avoid falling under its influence turns out to be nearly worthless. But five strategies to "de-bias" judgment have research support:

- *Consider alternative outcomes.* Actively considering alternatives, whether diagnoses or treatments, reduces unwarranted overconfidence and increases our humility.
- *Increase attention to usually ignored data.* Chief among such data are research findings, which help us to think realistically about probabilities and perhaps even to calculate likelihoods for our patients.
- *Minimize the role of memory.* Fallibility of recall should lead us to try to decrease our reliance on memory.
- *Use a disconfirmation strategy.* Instead of immediately searching for clinical information to support an initial hunch, search for information that would disconfirm it.

♦ *Rely on* **actuarial judgment** *when available.* As opposed to practitioner judgment alone, actuarial judgment relies on empirically
established statistical relationships between patient data and outcome. Hundreds of studies demonstrate the robust superiority of
actuarial over clinical judgment in making healthcare decisions.

Behavioral health practitioners have historically proved lousy at
gauging their clients' success and experiences of empathy, although
therapists frequently believe they do so with great accuracy
(Hannan et al., 2005). One meta-analysis found that client and therapist ratings of the quality of their therapeutic relationship were
correlated with a coefficient of only .33 on average (Tryon et al.,
2006). Therapists also do not judge very accurately who is doing
well in therapy; they tend to overestimate client gains and satisfaction (Lambert, 2013).

We can begin to evaluate ourselves better by asking questions
that force us to bypass heuristic biases, as suggested by Straus and
colleagues (2005):

♦ Have I asked myself any clinical questions lately?
♦ If so, have I asked well-formulated questions about both "foreground" and "background" issues (see Chapter 2)?
♦ Have I attempted to identify my own knowledge gaps and to frame
questions focused on those domains?
♦ Do I routinely note questions that occur to me in daily practice so
that I can follow up with research later?
♦ Are there better preventions, assessments, and treatments than
those I successfully employ now?

Once we get into the habit of routinely questioning ourselves about
our clinical work, the next step involves actively seeking answers. So
ask yourself the following:

♦ How often do I search the research literature?
♦ Do I know the best sources of current evidence for my profes-
sional discipline and patient population of interest?
♦ Do I have easy access to resources for finding the best available
evidence suited to my needs?
♦ Have I had success finding the research evidence I need?
♦ Have I become more efficient in my searches?
♦ Have I begun to critically appraise the evidence I discover?

♦ How do my searches and critical appraisals compare with those of respected colleagues who share my interest in seeking out and adopting the best EBPs?

♦ Have I become more critically sophisticated and accurate in applying to clinical practice what I have learned from the research?

If you ask yourself these questions, breaking free of heuristic biases whenever possible, you have essentially begun to audit your work—the next step in self-evaluation. An **audit** focuses on your performance in terms of outcomes. We will discuss application of audit principles to a clinic or program later in the chapter.

 Skill Exercise 10-2

Choose one of your recent clinical cases that has posed a challenge (e.g., in which the client did not progress or showed worsening symptoms). Set aside a half hour to search online for current evidence on the client's condition and context; use several of the filtered information sources presented in Chapter 3. Appraise how you might integrate the results you find into the client's care plan.

As an individual practitioner, you can (a) track patient outcomes, (b) check your work against evidence-based **practice guidelines**, and (c) compare patient outcomes with established **benchmarks** (when available). For example, one could measure treatment completion or dropout rates or use outcome measures (e.g., symptom changes in depression and anxiety measured with self-report instruments or observable behavioral indices such as days of sobriety or days missed from school or work). You might check yourself against the work of other practitioners at the same institution or as reported in the literature. You can also determine how your patient's progress compares with national benchmarks. (See Hunsley & Lee, 2007, for practical examples.)

Tracking Patient Outcomes

In the words of the APA Task Force on Evidence-Based Practice (2006, p. 285): "The application of research evidence to a given patient always involves probabilistic inferences. Therefore, ongoing monitoring of patient progress and adjustment of treatment as needed are essential [to EBPs]." We recommend that practitioners employ a four-pronged approach to collecting and using outcome data: patient self-report, ratings by other observers, quantifiable observable behaviors, and, when available, physiological data. We can link selection of the instruments directly to the individual circumstances of the client by using well-validated tools targeted to the patient's specific needs. (See Chapter 4 on accessing tests and measures, and see the December 2015 special issue of *Psychotherapy* on seven instruments for monitoring patient progress.)

Consider how this approach might apply to our three index patients. In Jonathon's case, we would typically track his ADHD and ODD symptoms by asking him and his parents to complete self-report checklists and other diagnostic instruments that assess their experience of his dysfunction. We might also ask for teacher reports and take care to address discrepancies among informants' ratings (De Los Reyes & Kazdin, 2004). If Jonathon were to undertake a course of neurofeedback (or electroencephalographic feedback) for his ADHD, then we would also seek to monitor the changes in the proportions of his brain waves. We could look for congruence of opinion and critically evaluate noncomporting data. For example, following multimodal intervention, it may turn out that parent and teacher reports reflect improvement. At the same time, Jonathon's acting-out behaviors decrease and his activity level moderates. If all of these changes occur with no concomitant brainwave changes, perhaps we should discard brainwave measurement as a meaningful outcome variable.

In Francesco's case, we might ask for self-report measures of life stresses, anxiety, and substance abuse. We might engage his primary-care physician to report on correlated physiological factors, for example, heart rate, blood pressure, or signs of hepatic disease. If available, we might also, with Francesco's consent, seek input from his family members or fellow workers regarding his alcohol consumption, emotional status, or days missed from work. And we might desire some concurrent monitoring of Francesco's blood alcohol levels with a breathalyzer or urine sample. Of course, we must take care to ascertain that the instruments we use are linguistically and culturally appropriate for Francesco, particularly if we wish to use comparative norms to track his progress.

In Annique's case, we can certainly rely on well-validated depression measures, but with her consent, we can also seek her spouse's and psychiatrist's views on her progress using standardized measures. We can also consider her absences from work, performance evaluations, use of alcohol or tobacco, sleeping, appetite, reports of somatic symptoms, and so on.

Because our three index patients, like the rest of the world, differ in age, sex, ethnicity, culture, socioeconomic class, and other characteristics, we must choose our assessment and outcome measures carefully, avoiding **arbitrary metrics**. Many psychological tests have arbitrary metrics but remain appropriate for testing theories (Blanton & Jaccard, 2006). For example, suppose we measure depression by asking someone, "How depressed do you feel on a scale of 1 to 7, where 1 equals not at all depressed and 7 equals totally depressed?" Such a scale might help us to track changes in that person's depression level over time, but a score of 5 on the scale has no absolute meaning apart from any arbitrary criteria or cut points that we set. The same factors or symptoms that contribute to one person's rating of 5 might lead a different person to offer a rating of 4 or 6. In addition, patients may intentionally under- or overreport levels of distress, for a wide range of individual motives.

Behavioral health and addiction research has traditionally relied heavily on such metrics, and investigators may find themselves unable to determine whether patients receiving EBPs have improved in their daily lives or have changed in significant ways apart from the arbitrary metrics. What if Jonathon's parents rate him as improved on instrument norms but his teacher finds him unmanageable in class? Suppose Francesco reports less anxiety than the test manual specifies for the average Latino male, but he took the test while intoxicated? Perhaps Annique will report improved quality of life according to the test manual despite the fact that her spouse witnesses continued chronic tearfulness and sleep disturbance. Annique may worry that the therapist she has come to like and trust will feel badly if she does not report "doing better." In translating EBP case by case, we must better connect arbitrary measures to real-world referents (Kazdin, 2006).

As all practitioners know, assessing patient outcome and treatment success usually proves far more complicated than can be conveyed by a single, global category of "improved" or "not improved." In reviewing research, we would categorize this as a **criterion problem**: What criteria are most appropriate for determining effective treatment, and who should decide? We embrace the tripartite view of mental health outcomes (Strupp & Hadley, 1977): the individual patient's perspective, the family and societal perspective, and the treating clinician's perspective. The same individual may qualify simultaneously as cured, improved, or deteriorating depending upon the criteria used. Similarly, the same treatment may simultaneously qualify as a successful evidence-based approach, an unsuccessful evidence-based approach, or a non-evidence-based approach depending upon the person setting the criteria.

We have thus far discussed the evaluation of patient outcomes largely in terms of symptom improvement at the end of a course of treatment. However, experienced clinicians know that we must consider evaluating the ongoing process, including the treatment relationship. We recommend assessing patient satisfaction with treatment, monitoring patient progress, and making mid-course treatment corrections or adjustments as needed.

Research has underscored the effectiveness of systematically seeking patients' feedback as a way to materially improve the success of therapy. Meta-analyses of RCTs (Lambert, 2012; Norcross, 2011) demonstrated that collecting feedback from patients periodically throughout treatment is positively associated with therapy outcome ($d = 0.49 - 0.70$) and reduced by about half the chances of at-risk patients experiencing deterioration. We can improve outcomes by detecting deterioration early and altering the course of treatment.

The EBP moral: Regularly and proactively request real-time feedback from clients on their response to the therapy relationship. Privilege the *client's* experience of the treatment relationship and success, not the therapist's perspective. The benefits of doing so include empowering clients, promoting explicit collaboration, allowing for midtherapy adjustments as needed, and enhancing the success of treatment (S. D. Miller et al., 2005).

The data—both empirical and clinical—on regularly collecting feedback from patients appear compelling. Many clinicians will tell us, "Of course, I do this stuff with my patients." However, the research indicates that they do *not* do such assessment regularly. Even when clinicians solicit such information, they often do not do so *explicitly*—instead, they intuit or infer. And they often prove inaccurate when guessing or inferring. Some clinicians find it awkward to broach discussion of the relationship with the client and may blame the patient for any disappointments or ruptures. Evidence-based practice demands that we follow the evidence on how to collect feedback, conceptualize patient dissatisfaction as a mutual problem, and hold paramount the patient's experience of treatment.

Checking Your Work Against Practice Guidelines

Individual practitioners can compare their performance against the guidelines introduced earlier in this book (see especially Chapter 3). The most exhaustive listings of healthcare guidelines probably appear at the National Guideline Clearinghouse (www.guideline.gov) and the National Institute for Health and Clinical Excellence (www.nice.org.uk).

Comparing Patient Outcomes With Established Benchmarks

Using Jonathon as an example, we have already noted how a practitioner can track patient outcomes using self-ratings, parent ratings, and teacher ratings. We could also compare our ability to retain the family in treatment against dropout rates reported in the literature, retention rates for colleagues at our institution, or rates for other, similar patients in our practice. Then we could compare our treatment of Jonathon against established professional guidelines.

Jonathon's pediatrician, for example, could check the management of his asthma against standards for inhaled medication (see, e.g., www.nice.org.uk/guidance/TA38?c=91527) and for the potential drug interactions in his ADHD treatment plan (see, e.g., pediatrics.aappublications.org/content/108/4/1033). Regarding the ADHD, the American Academy of Pediatrics would recommend that Jonathon's primary-care physician attend to five foci: (1) establishing a treatment program that recognizes ADHD as a chronic condition; (2) ensuring that the treating clinician works in collaboration with the parents, child, and school personnel while specifying target outcomes; (3) recommending stimulant medication, behavior therapy, or both to improve target outcomes; (4) if the selected management program does not meet target outcomes, re-evaluating the original diagnosis, using all appropriate treatments, considering adherence to the treatment plan, and considering the presence of coexisting problems; (5) providing a systematic follow-up for the child directed at the target outcomes and using information gathered from the child, parents, and teachers.

Obviously, a behavioral health practitioner could follow a similar plan in close concert with the primary-care physician. This model tracks well with the diagnostic and decision trees illustrated in Figures 8.1 and 8.2.

Evaluating the Program or Organization

In addition to evaluating your own use of EBPs, it is important to examine the group, program, or organization within which you practice. Organizational structures may create barriers to change that prove as or more difficult to alter than the behavior of individual practitioners.

One strategy for auditing groups or institutions involves implementing a plan–do–check–act cycle (Straus et al., 2005). Typical barriers encountered in group practice or institutional settings include the disparate levels of acceptance (different stages of change) and varying levels of education and training among different personnel. Professionals responsible for different activities—for example, intake, screening, evaluation, assignment, record-keeping, and in-service training—can inhibit change.

In the "plan" phase of the cycle, as its name suggests, we make plans for implementing EBPs within the organization, including addressing institutional barriers. Some types of EBPs will prove easier to implement than others. In-service training programs, continuing-education opportunities, focused case conferences, and journal clubs can all contribute to upgrading practitioner competence (see Chapter 11 for a full discussion of enhancing implementation).

After initial planning and targeting the barriers to implementation, the next phase of the audit will involve "doing." We can conceptualize this as a pilot period of testing the ability to change. Ideally, this phase will involve solid efforts to measure change by establishing initial or historical base rates and then reviewing comparison data after attempting the new model. We follow this period with "checking" activity aimed at answering the following questions: Did the expected changes occur? Do patient outcome data seem congruent with administrative systems data? What worked? What did not work? Why?

In the final, "act" step of the organizational practice audit, we look at how to systematize and extend the gains documented in the review of the pilot data, or we revisit our original plan in an effort to fix the parts that did not work as anticipated. Often this will involve adapting to the human element of the equation. For example, we may find that some practitioners have resisted changing or otherwise failed to adapt their ways of working. Introduction of benchmark comparisons, particularly from external sources, or practice guidelines can help overcome resistance and motivate change.

Alternatively, we may find that the idealized EBP model does not fit our population well. Jonathon's parents, for example, may have significant difficulty in following the clinician's suggestions consistently, nullifying the effect of our best efforts at parent management training. Francesco's lack of health insurance and the agency's inability to offer reduced-fee or pro bono services may result in his dropping out of treatment. Annique may become acutely suicidal and require hospitalization before her treatment with cognitive–behavior therapy and new medication get underway.

Successful application of the audit will require careful, objective analysis of any failures and modification of planning to address root issues in a revised series of steps. Optimal success occurs when this cycle of planning, doing, checking, and acting becomes routine.

Evaluating the Profession

Healthcare professionals must actively define and implement EBPs in a manner that best serves their clientele and professional values. Otherwise we will find ourselves floundering in the wake created by the other health professions' inexorable movement in that direction. Either we participate in EBPs or others will commandeer the process at our expense.

We must consider whether our educational and training programs tend to create uninvolved professionals or colleagues actively engaged in continuous quality improvement. Early debate and dialogue on EBP among mental health professionals seemed to revolve around fears of criticism and narcissistic injury: "Your criticisms about the way I practice just aren't fair, because . . ." Books on the topic tended toward the descriptive and interpretive, aimed at informing practitioners and defusing tensions (Norcross et al., 2006a). We recognize, however, that passive dissemination of EBP materials will prove insufficient to bring about real change (see Chapter 11).

This book represents movement from the preparation stage to the action stage of EBPs by providing practical, how-to applications.

We hope to trigger change in individual behavior that will ultimately evoke broader professional change in behavioral health and addictions practice. Medicine has seen this occur as insurers and government agencies begin to designate preferred providers. For example, some hospitals with better surgical outcomes for specific procedures have won preferred-provider designations from some payers.

Of course, debate will center on the appropriateness of outcome variables. Most of us would prefer reduced symptoms, absence of side effects, and improved quality of life as outcomes, but we fear that some payers in the healthcare industry will value cost of services more highly than patient-centered variables. Healthcare costs decrease when surgical outcomes go well and no additional hospitalizations or expensive tests are required. However, subsequent healthcare costs also drop when the patient dies in surgery.

Managed-care organizations and other third-party payers have begun to deploy their own outcome measures for subscribers utilizing medical, mental health, and substance abuse services. Some payers refer to using these measures as a "quality assurance plan," but others describe it as a **pay for performance (P4P)** plan intended to improve the quality of healthcare. The P4P programs yield valuable outcome data but also pose significant implementation concerns (Bachman, 2006) and ethical challenges (e.g., collection of large databases filled with confidential information that patients may prefer not to disclose to their insurance companies). In addition, outcome measures designed by and for third-party payers will likely raise the same questions highlighted in our opening chapter: What data will best validate the preferred outcome for which patients?

Risk Management and Evidence-Based Practices

Risk management uses retrospective evaluation for the prospective assessment of practice hazards. Risk management may involve addressing ethical violations, carelessness, simple errors, or even unfortunate outcomes without any actual negligence. The key to basic risk management is understanding standards of care.

From a legal perspective, the clinician must possess and use the knowledge, skill, and care ordinarily possessed by members of the profession in good standing. From an ethical perspective, meeting the **standard of care** means adhering to the prevailing professional judgment of peers engaged in similar activities in similar circumstances, given the knowledge the clinician had or should have had at the time. From a risk management perspective, EBP, when properly implemented, tends to lower one's risk of an adverse incident.

Since EBP is frequently adapted to individual patients, how much risk does adaptation or innovation with established protocols incur? Conservative decision-making often proves safest and most faithful to established practice, but one can quite reasonably take prudent risks when they offer a good probability of improving treatment outcomes without substantially increasing the risk of harm. Prudent risk-taking involves drawing on collegial consultation and producing good documentation. Such steps enable the clinician to demonstrate that he or she provided good care, behaved as a competent, prudent professional, and engaged in ethically sound conduct, consistent with the law and the standard of care.

As an example of prudent risk-taking, let us consider Annique's return to psychotherapy. As in treating any depressed patient, the usual standard of care would include inquiring about suicidal ideation. Suppose that Annique's therapist asks this question, and Annique reports that she has "thought about it from time to time." This response would trigger additional questions from the prudent practitioner. Let us assume that further inquiry reveals the following: Annique has no history of suicide attempts, has not formulated a plan, has articulated the importance of and delight she takes in interacting with her young grandchild, and has forged a positive alliance with the therapist. In this context, one could reasonably rate her risk of self-harm as low and put aside any thoughts of seeking inpatient treatment.

Another example, focused on Francesco, might involve the clinician making a collateral referral to a community agency providing blue-collar job placement. Some practitioners might wonder: "Will I offend Francesco by suggesting he ought to be looking for work? Will he feel uncomfortable about returning to therapy if he does not follow the suggestion? Will his anxiety increase if the program rejects him?" All of these questions do raise potential risks, but they are risks worth taking. By making such a referral, the clinician conveys an interest in addressing Francesco's sources of anxiety and demonstrates a concern that reaches beyond the traditional domain of the therapeutic relationship.

Keep in mind that the greatest risk may be to stop taking any risks—with the end result that EBPs may stifle creative, innovative, and nimble practice. Clinicians must remain responsive. The challenge involves blending innovation with empiricism. Either extreme—too much risk or too little restraint, on the one hand, or being too rule and research bound, on the other—probably harms patients.

Mistakes Versus Negligence

People cannot avoid making mistakes, but a mistake does not equal negligence. Practitioners can and will make "judgment call" errors. We need not attain perfection, but we must strive to be at least "good enough" clinicians (Bennett et al., 2007).

The two terms that signify the most risk are *departure from standard of care* and *gross negligence*. A practice representing **departure from standard of care** is one that many practitioners would not do, while **gross negligence** represents an extreme departure from usual professional conduct. In this regard, implementing EBP as a result of cogent reasoning and thoughtful consultation will tend to insulate the practitioner from risks associated with lawsuits and licensing board complaints alleging negligence.

For a lawsuit to succeed, a plaintiff's attorney must generally prove the **four Ds of legal liability**: *d*ereliction of *d*uty leading *d*irectly to *d*amages (Bennett et al., 2007; Knapp et al., 2013):

♦ A *duty* applies when the clinician agrees to provide services to the patient and they begin to work together in a professional relationship.
♦ *Dereliction* implies a breach of duty and, by extension, negligence. Dereliction or negligence may include acts of commission or acts of omission. As an example of an act of commission, we can imagine that Jonathon attempts to leap from the therapist's desk, breaking a prized clock, and the angry clinician, trying to restrain Jonathon, grabs his arm and causes him to fall and sustain a fracture. An act of omission might be Annique's therapist's failing during three sessions to inquire whether she has had any thoughts of suicide, only to learn that she has subsequently killed herself.
♦ Attorneys usually attempt to demonstrate *direct* causation using a doctrine of proximal cause. In so doing they seek to prove that the clinician's negligence led directly (or contributed proximally) to the harm suffered by the patient.

◆ To document *damages,* the plaintiff's attorney will use invoices (e.g., hospital bills or fees paid to subsequent therapists) or experts (e.g., a forensic economist to testify about the lifetime earnings lost due to Annique's death or the toll on her spouse for loss of consortium).

You can take charge of your practice and reduce the likelihood of a lawsuit (Bennett et al., 2007; Knapp et al., 2013; Woody, 2013) by

◆ maintaining a working knowledge of ethics codes and legal standards governing practice;
◆ conservatively evaluating your competence to perform;
◆ maintaining intellectual, technical, and emotional competence;
◆ documenting your actions and consulting with peers;
◆ keeping your knowledge up to date;
◆ preventing financial considerations from dominating your decision-making;
◆ making modest professional representations;
◆ implementing a risk management system; and
◆ screening clients to eliminate (or at least foresee) undue risks.

At times you may have to consider termination of a client whose behavior becomes risky or prevents you from delivering optimal care. For example, if Jonathon has failed to improve after rigorous efforts with an EBP for externalizing behaviors, and his parents still decline to consider medication, you should consider the ethical obligation to terminate or refer a client who has not benefited from your efforts. A similar situation might occur if Annique ceased taking her medication and experienced a worsening depression despite your best therapeutic efforts.

Liability and Innovation

If we only conduct EBP, how will innovation occur? What standards apply when attempting to assess the relationship between liability and innovation in patient care? One clear standard involves what courts regard as scientifically acceptable evidence.

The ruling in *Daubert v. Merrell Dow Pharmaceuticals, Inc.* (1993) provides some valuable guidance. Prior to that case, the standard for introducing scientific evidence in court was *general acceptance*, sometimes known as the Frye standard, dating from 1923. The *Daubert* case focused on the admissibility of novel scientific evidence in federal courts and firmly established the judge as a gatekeeper to ensure that any evidence considered in court has both relevance and reliability.

In the *Daubert* case, the families of two boys born with birth defects sued Merrell Dow Pharmaceuticals, claiming that the drug doxylamine succinate (Bendectin), used to treat morning sickness, caused the defects. Merrell Dow's expert witness planned to testify that no published scientific studies demonstrated a link between Bendectin and birth defects. Plaintiffs' counsel submitted expert evidence of its own suggesting that Bendectin could potentially cause human birth defects. However, that evidence came from laboratory studies using cell cultures and laboratory animals, reanalysis of other published studies, and methodologies that had not yet gained acceptance within the general scientific community. Furthermore, the court seemed skeptical because the plaintiffs' evidence appeared to have been generated solely for the purpose of the litigation. Without that questionable evidence, the court doubted that the plaintiffs could prove at trial that the Bendectin had in fact caused the birth defects. In essence, the court doubted the methodological validity and generalizability of the evidence used to prove the drug caused the problem.

(Parenthetically, this case also provides a good example of a scientific question for which we could not conduct a true RCT. After all, we could not ethically use random assignment of nauseous pregnant women to a Bendectin treatment condition if we had any reason to suspect birth defects might result.)

The *Daubert* standard has three key provisions:

1. Expert testimony must have a scientific basis.
2. The scientific knowledge must assist the trier of fact (the judge or jury) in understanding or determining a fact at issue in the case.
3. The judge makes the determination regarding whether the scientific knowledge would indeed assist the trier of fact by ruling whether the reasoning or methodology underlying the testimony stands as scientifically valid and whether that reasoning or methodology can properly be applied to the facts at issue.

The judge's preliminary assessment can focus on whether something has undergone testing, whether an idea has passed scientific peer review or achieved publication in scientific journals, falsifiability of data and error rates involved in a technique, and even, in certain circumstances, general acceptance. The judicial decision focuses on methodology and principles, not the ultimate conclusions generated. Federal courts have applied the standards in *Daubert* strictly, and they have succeeded in excluding "junk science" or "pseudoscience" as well as techniques that qualify as merely experimental.

These standards can guide the efforts of clinicians planning an innovation or EBP adaptation in their practice by suggesting criteria for anticipating criticism or legal challenges. Demonstrating that one's approach, whether a treatment method, prevention program, or assessment measure, has a grounding in valid and reliable science, passes peer review, or has won general acceptance by peer practitioners indicates that it has likely passed a legal acceptance threshold (at least as evidence).

In a subsequent "junk science" case (*Kumho Tire Co., Ltd. v. Carmichael*, 1999), the courts ultimately excluded a technician's testimony that an exploding tire must have caused an accident because he could find no other reason for the tire's failure. In other words, the technician asserted a causal relationship based on an absence of data. The message for potential innovators is to predicate new approaches on proven foundations, collect pilot data on interventions suspected of being effective, and consider sources of error when attempting to generalize from population to population or setting to setting. Once again, the key to acceptance of science in the courtroom is reliable and valid scientific knowledge.

For a concrete example, suppose Francesco establishes a solid therapeutic alliance with you, a new clinician who has effectively used EBPs to help bring his anxiety and substance abuse under control. Francesco's referral to the job training program has won him steady employment, with health insurance, at a new automobile assembly plant across the state. Francesco wants to continue in treatment to consolidate his gains, but he says he trusts only you. After all, you've helped turn his life around. He wants to continue treatment with you by telephone after he relocates.

We may not have an RCT to demonstrate the efficacy of continuity of treatment by telephone, nor will we likely ever have one. Even if we could set up a scientific study of this practice, Francesco would never agree to randomization, and neither would other patients who have solid alliances with their clinicians. One could easily advance ethical arguments against such a study. We do know, however, that Francesco has a therapeutic relationship of proven effectiveness and apparently strong motivation to persist along the same lines. We can certainly make a reasonable argument in favor of attempting the innovative follow-up treatment.

Ethics and Evidence-Based Practices

The key ethical considerations in EBP revolve around matters of competence, consent, and public statements. More specifically, the central EBP elements of all professional ethics focus on fundamental questions of practitioner competence, patients' sense of autonomy or self-determination as afforded via consent, and the accuracy of public statements about our services. The American Psychological Association's ethics code (APA, 2010a) covers these issues well; thus we shall use it as an exemplar for the various codes of behavioral health and addictions professions. Table 10.3 demonstrates the close correspondence between EBPs and practitioners' ethical obligations to patients.

 The book's companion website contains hyperlinks to the ethics codes of the major behavioral health and addiction associations in the United States.

Competence

As a starting point, we must remain mindful that the ethics codes demand that clinicians have both the scientific and professional skills needed to serve their patients. Our choice of a treatment method versus other potential methods must have a foundation in scientific evidence. According to the APA ethics code (2010a),

TABLE 10.3 Relation of Evidence-Based Practice (EBP) to Ethical Principles

Obligation to patients	Relation to EBP
Help patients and avoid harm (beneficence and nonmaleficence)	Enabling access to clinical and policy-related research findings optimizes likelihood of success and minimizes risk of harm.
Optimize self-determination (autonomy)	Involving patients in clinical decision-making regarding risks, benefits, and alternatives in the context of evidence provides more meaningful choices.
Respect and integrity (fidelity)	Minimizing coercion, understanding and respecting patient preferences, avoiding biases and stereotypes, and adapting EBPs to suit human differences promotes respect and maintains integrity.
Competence	Having the knowledge and skill to provide evidence-based care requires keeping up to date with practice-related knowledge and knowing where to find it.
Accountability	Monitoring progress by seeking ongoing feedback during the course of treatment assures accountability.
Social justice	Advocating for one's patients in the face of economic, policy, and health system changes can be more effective when practices are buttressed with evidence of effectiveness.
Lifelong learning	Helping practitioners value lifelong learning and providing the necessary tools to stay up to date are critical components of EBP.
Research value	Assuring that research addresses topics and questions of real-world value to patients and practitioners is central to EBP.

Note: Adapted from Gambrill (2012).

"Psychologists undertake ongoing efforts to develop and maintain their competence" (section 2.03) and "Psychologists' work is based upon established scientific and professional knowledge of the discipline" (section 2.04).

Clinicians have an obligation to work only within the boundaries of their competence based on education, training, supervised experience, consultation, study, or professional experience. This obligation requires us to remain cautious when evaluating our own expertise. In conducting a new EBP, a professional would need to acquire competence in it, not merely passing familiarity. Reading a treatment manual alone would probably not constitute sufficient preparation to establish competence. In addition to the strategies and tactics associated with particular approaches, the clinician needs a thorough understanding of psychopathology, diagnostic assessment, and individual differences to properly assess and treat the patient. True competence requires a degree of self-awareness that helps us feel confident of what we know while recognizing what we do not know.

In some situations, requirements for additional knowledge and integration skills might apply. Each of our index cases, for example, displays somatic features that require the clinician to have, or acquire through consultation, some medical knowledge. Jonathon may experience an exacerbation of agitation, manifesting hyperactivity as a side effect of albuterol, his asthma medication. Francesco may suffer from medical symptoms related to his history of alcohol abuse. Hormonal changes associated with Annique's menopausal condition may contribute to her mood disorder.

Another subset of competence involves the ability to tailor EBP to the needs of individuals (see also Chapter 9). Where our scientific or professional knowledge establishes that a particular patient differs in factors associated with age, gender, race, ethnicity, culture, religion, sexual orientation, disability, language, or socioeconomic status from the patients described in the research on the EBP in question, we must stand prepared to adapt the EBP to reflect the patient's needs, values, and preferences. This obligation may require us to obtain the training, experience, consultation, or supervision necessary to ensure the competence of our services or to make an appropriate referral.

Skill Exercise 10-3

Current estimates of the half-life of knowledge acquired in the doctoral education of psychologists run less than nine years (Koocher & Keith-Spiegel, 2016). Design a plan for keeping your knowledge base up to date by addressing three questions: (1) What steps will I take to remain current on best practices for the population(s) I treat most often? (2) How can I assure myself that I will critically appraise my knowledge level? (3) How will I regularly integrate updated knowledge into my practice?

At the same time, we must recognize that no professional will know everything and that the patient's ideal match may not sit waiting for a call. Suppose that Francesco's first language was Spanish, Annique's was Creole, and Jonathon's was Serbo-Croatian. Suppose they are immigrants, perhaps even undocumented, or that they are witnesses to or victims of violence. Now suppose that they present in your office with a moderate level of English proficiency seeking help, and no other behavioral health or substance abuse professional lives within a reasonable commuting distance. You have a solid knowledge of EBPs that apply to their problems, but you have never treated anyone exactly like them before. If you stand prepared to listen and learn from your patients and their families (or to consult with others who have special knowledge you lack), you may well have the ability to apply EBPs in ways likely to generalize to and benefit these clients. Doing so remains ethically appropriate if you obtain the client's consent after acknowledging any limitations or constraints.

Consent

When practitioners conduct any professional service, they must obtain the consent of the patient(s). Note from the outset that we have not inserted the adjective *informed* in front of the noun *consent*. Doing so would create a tautology or redundancy, since consent must, by definition, constitute a knowing and voluntary act. The accepted standard holds that before they can give consent, people must have all of the information that might reasonably influence their willingness to participate in the task at hand. The information must be in a form (language, format, and reading level) that enables them to reasonably grasp it. In addition, the recipient of the information must have the legal authority and personal competence (e.g., not comatose or severely cognitively impaired) to make and give voice to the decision.

One can only give consent for oneself, so a parent or legal guardian who authorizes treatment for a child or ward has given *permission* (sometimes called *proxy consent* by ethicists). When the patient lacks the legal competence to give consent because of age or mental impairment, practitioners must nevertheless provide an appropriate explanation, seek the patient's assent, and consider the patient's preferences and best interests.

Competent patients have a right to refuse treatment in most circumstances. Exceptions apply to some patients who pose an urgent threat to themselves or to others or who are incarcerated. Suppose that we recommend a trial of stimulant medication for Jonathon, disulfiram (Antabuse) for Francesco, and lithium for Annique. Now suppose that the adult patients and Jonathon's parents, concerned about potential side effects, say, "No, thank you." Some patients may raise religious objections to specific medical or behavioral interventions—for example, Jehovah's Witnesses (objections to blood products), Seventh-day Adventists (objections to hypnosis), and Christian Scientists (preference for spiritual intervention). Conversely, Jonathon may object to some aspects of a treatment program, such as "time-outs" or medication, but his parents have the right to trump his preferences.

Consent with respect to EBP involves active efforts to inform participants of the nature of treatment, potential side effects (if any), and alternative treatments. Enthusiastic proponents of particular EBPs may feel so positively about their interventions that they do not take adequate time to fully discuss the treatment plan with the patient. In almost every case, taking the time to discuss the treatment will actively engage the client in the treatment process while allowing opportunities for any reservations to emerge. Viewing the consent process as part of forging a therapeutic relationship rather than an "ethical chore" will prove highly effective.

 Skill Exercise 10-4

Consider the research-supported treatments you would want to use in treating one of our index patients. Now imagine that the patient has been raised in an unusual lifestyle or practices an unconventional religion that leads him or her to object to the recommended treatment plan. State the objection and draft the language you would use to discuss this issue with the patient, giving consideration to his or her perspectives, beliefs, culture, and preferences as well as any alternative treatments you would consider.

Advertising and Public Statements

A final important ethical consideration entails avoiding false or deceptive public statements about our work, including touting the merits of particular EBPs or criticizing other practitioners. In this context, public statements include paid or unpaid advertising, product endorsements, licensing applications, brochures, printed matter, directory listings, personal resumes, media comments, statements in legal proceedings, oral presentations, and published materials.

Clinicians should not knowingly make public statements that directly or indirectly convey false, deceptive, or fraudulent content. Examples include the following:

♦ "Scientific research demonstrates that my treatment is the most effective for anxiety disorders" (an assertion highly unlikely to be accurate without numerous qualifying statements).

♦ "Those cognitive–behavioral therapies do not produce any lasting changes and almost always result in relapse or symptom substitution" (yet research demonstrates that many such therapies frequently can and do yield lasting beneficial changes).

♦ One of our personal favorites: A clinician—we'll call him "Jones"—tacked a letter onto the front of a well-known EBP acronym and touted "JCBT—a breakthrough therapy for depression!" It seems that "JCBT" stood for "Jones cognitive–behavioral therapy," meaning cognitive–behavioral therapy as performed by him. Unless you asked, you might never learn what the "J" stood for or that he had no data whatever to support his claim.

Remember: Ethical practice in EBP (as a subset of behavioral health and substance abuse practice) centers on clinician competence, full consent, and accurate public statements supportable by hard data.

Key Terms

actuarial judgment
arbitrary metrics
audit
benchmarks
criterion problem
departure from standard of care
four Ds of legal liability

gross negligence
heuristics
pay for performance (P4P)
practice guidelines
risk management
standard of care

Recommended Readings and Websites

Cone, J. D. (2000). *Evaluating outcomes: Empirical tools for effective practice.* Washington, DC: American Psychological Association.

Farmer, R. F., & Chapman, A. L. (2016). *Behavioral interventions in cognitive behavior therapy: Practical guidance for putting theory into action.* Washington, DC: American Psychological Association.

Gambrill, E. (2012). *Critical thinking in clinical practice: Improving the quality of judgments and decisions* (3rd ed.). Hoboken, NJ: Wiley.

Hunsley, J., & Lee, C. M. (2007). Research-informed benchmarks for psychological treatments: Efficacy studies, effectiveness studies, and beyond. *Professional Psychology: Research and Practice, 38,* 21–33.

Kahneman, D., & Tversky, A. (Eds.). (2000). *Choices, values, and frames.* New York, NY: Cambridge University Press.

Knapp, S., Younggren, J. N., VandeCreek, L., Harris, E., and Martin, J. N. (2013). Assessing and managing risk in psychological practice: An individualized approach (2nd ed.). Bethesda, MD: The Trust.

Koocher, G. P., & Keith-Spiegel, P. (2016). *Ethical principles in psychology and the mental health professions: Standards and cases* (4th ed.). New York, NY: Oxford University Press.

Mentz, R. J., Hernandez, A. F., Berdan, L. G., Rorick, T., O'Brien, E. C., Ibarra, J. C., . . . Peterson, E. D. (2016). Good clinical practice guidance and pragmatic clinical trials: Balancing the best of both worlds. *Circulation, 133*(9), 872–880.

National Guideline Clearinghouse, www.guideline.gov

National Institute for Health and Clinical Excellence, www.nice.org.uk

Royse, D., Thyer, B., & Padgett, D. (2015). *Program evaluation: An introduction to an evidence-based approach.* Belmont, CA: Cengage.

Youngstrom, E. A., Choukas-Bradley, S., Calhoun, C. D., & Jensen-Doss, A. (2015). Clinical guide to the evidence-based assessment approach to diagnosis and treatment. *Cognitive and Behavioral Practice, 22*(1), 20–35.

11

Disseminating, Teaching, and Implementing Evidence-Based Practices

S CIENTISTS ARE ENAMORED WITH, PERHAPS EVEN addicted to, discovery. Not so much with the implementation of their discoveries, however. Commentators have characterized the gulf between discovery of a research-supported treatment, prevention, test, or other intervention and its implementation as "the valley of death," "a clogged pipeline," the "research–practice gap," and the "culture wars."

Moving research evidence from science to service, from the lab bench to the bedside, poses a thorny problem for evidence-based practices (EBPs) across all of healthcare. Of course, slow or begrudging adoption is not unique to behavioral health and addictions; sluggish diffusion bedevils most fields, ranging from education and agriculture to business and communication (Rogers, 2003).

Translation(al) research inclusively refers to the process of successfully moving research-supported discoveries into established practice and policy. As a celebrated quote from Göethe puts it: "Knowing is not enough; we must apply. Willing is not enough;

we must do." Or as Yoda said: "Do or do not. There is no try." Translation (or translational) research includes many complex components of this process, but prominently research into disseminating, teaching, and implementing EBPs.

The international juggernaut of EBPs has now affected every healthcare profession and has increasingly found its way into education and training programs. Accompanying this progress we find a cornucopia of online materials and tools for teaching EBPs (and evidence-based medicine, or EBM); simply try any search engine and you will instantly locate hundreds of examples. One can now complete an entire course, secure a certificate, and even obtain a graduate degree in EBP.

Ironically, despite jumping onto the EBP bandwagon, many of the training tutorials and courses offer no research evidence for their own effectiveness in teaching or implementing EBPs! Having learned from their experience, we begin this chapter with synopses of the empirical research on predicting adoption of EBPs and the barriers to adoption and implementation of EBPs. We then turn our attention to specific methods for disseminating, teaching, and implementing EBPs.

 Skill Exercise 11-1

Type "training in evidence based practice" into your favorite Internet search engine, hit Enter, blink twice, and watch tens of thousands of websites appear, covering virtually every imaginable profession. Scan the entries and possibilities. Then, type "training in evidence based (your profession or specialty)" and see what's offered in your particular field. Can you locate any research evidence for the effectiveness of the training programs that come up in teaching EBPs?

Who Is Drawn Toward EBPs?

A small but growing stream of empirical studies has examined the predictors of practitioners' propensity to use EBP and EBM (e.g., Aarons, 2006; Gotham, 2004; Jensen-Doss et al., 2009; Jette et al., 2003; Klimes-Dougan et al., 2009; Nelson & Steele, 2007; Pagoto et al., 2007; Sheehan et al., 2007). The studies uniformly find that the majority of practitioners continue to rely foremost on the traditional (i.e., non-EBP) information sources of clinical experience, peer opinions, and textbooks. Far fewer practitioners look first to practice guidelines, Cochrane Reviews, and related EBP sources. Across studies, the significant predictors of adopting EBPs or expressing positive attitudes toward them include the practitioner's

◆ desire to learn and openness to new practices;
◆ graduate training in EBP, such as taking an EBP class;
◆ quality of the clinical training received in previous EBPs;
◆ favorable opinion of treatment research;
◆ perceived receptivity of the workplace toward EBPs;
◆ supervisors' modeling of and reinforcement for using EBPs;
◆ perception that EBP can be used in daily practice without detracting from clinical productivity (practicality);
◆ employment in (or planning a career in) research;
◆ younger age (the only consistently predictive demographic variable);
◆ personality traits of openness, conscientiousness, and low neuroticism; and
◆ more formal education and attainment of a higher degree.

While practitioner variables exert a strong influence, so too do organizational and economic factors; these, however, generally prove more difficult to detect in survey studies. Organizations that facilitate learning EBPs by providing release time and in-house training, for example, are more likely to sustain EBPs than organizations primarily concerned with short-term cost containment. Practice settings with high burnout rates seem unlikely to incubate EBPs, which often require stepping outside one's comfort zone and acquiring new skills with the support and consultation of colleagues (Addis, 2002).

Negative predictors of EBP largely comprise the converse of the preceding list. These include advanced practitioner age, high percentage of time spent in direct patient care, negative opinions about treatment research, lack of access to EBP resources at work, and absence of explicit training in EBP. Indeed, the principal barrier appears not to be skepticism but rather a lack of knowledge of EBP and its core skills.

 Skill Exercise 11-2

And what of your own attitude toward EBPs? Take the Evidence-Based Practice Attitude Scale (EBPAS), available at no charge from the author (at psychiatry.ucsd. edu/research/casrc/resources/Documents/EBPAS-50.pdf or contact Dr. Gregory Aarons at gaarons@ucsd. edu). Compare your scores to the national norms published in Aarons et al. (2010). How do you stack up to your colleagues on the four subscales?

Barriers to Adoption and Implementation of EBPs

Research results and common sense tell us that practitioners' attitudes toward EBPs constitute a huge factor in adopting and implementing them. Clinicians frequently complain of difficulty in meeting client needs without deviating from the research-supported protocol. They worry about how to build in flexibility while preserving fidelity (see Chapters 8 and 9). Individual inertia, dearth of local training, and reluctance to change challenge all new developments. In the absence of an institutional affiliation or library resources, access to the online databases is prohibitively expensive. In one study of independent practitioners, the strongest predictor of unwillingness to obtain EBP training involved the amount of time and the cost required for the training (Stewart et al., 2011).

But the organization and leadership pose barriers as well. Systemically, the lack of agency resources for training and the extensive costs associated with changing clinical practices are obstacles frequently mentioned by community clinicians. Leadership failures prove a key factor: leadership in partnering with staff and community groups, leadership in innovation adoption, leadership in modeling EBPs, and leadership in maintaining EBPs (when colleagues and agency support wane). In fact, systematic reviews of successful, large-scale implementation programs found that they almost universally (a) required agency support, (b) involved early adoption, (c) engaged heterogeneous stakeholders, and (d) conducted a structured needs assessment (McHugh & Barlow, 2012). Long-term EBP implementation begins with the leaders of organizations.

Three Training Steps

Getting clinicians to use EBPs in daily practice consists of three distinct but overlapping training steps. The first step is **dissemination**, which entails raising awareness of EBP resources, particularly the supporting research evidence, and their availability. Clinicians need to know about the availability, accessibility, and utility of resources. The second step entails teaching the requisite core EBP skills to competence. Clinicians need to know how to do EBP. And the third step is **implementation**, which involves getting practitioners to routinely use evidence in practice. Each step implicates different strategies and different stakeholders.

Disseminating Evidence-Based Practices

Reviews of the empirical research on dissemination of EBPs uniformly conclude that passive dissemination of EBP materials by itself exerts no significant effect on practitioner behavior (e.g., National Implementation Research Network [NIRN], 2005; NHS Centre for Reviews and Dissemination, 1999). In a systematic review of 102 trials on methods to improve healthcare practice, for example, the authors (Oxman et al., 1995) concluded that dissemination-only activities result in little or no behavior change. Passive dissemination of EBPs is not an EBP!

The empirical findings have directed EBP training efforts in crucial ways. For one, dissemination of information alone does *not* result in positive implementation outcomes (changes in practitioner behavior) or treatment outcomes (benefits to consumers). Only the naive will believe that when research information becomes available, busy clinicians will access, appraise, and then routinely apply it. Dissemination-alone strategies have proved largely discredited and should be abandoned. For another, practitioner training proves more effective than information dissemination alone (NIRN, 2005). Thus we should

0

focus on actively teaching the EBP skills—to which we now turn—
and then on systems implementation—to which we turn shortly.

Teaching Evidence-Based Practices

Several sets of researchers have painstakingly reviewed the thousands of empirical studies on effective teaching in higher education.
They have converged on several conclusions. Good EBP in higher
education (Chickering & Gamson, 1987)

◆ encourages contacts between students and faculty,
◆ develops reciprocity and cooperation among students,
◆ uses active learning techniques,
◆ gives prompt feedback,
◆ emphasizes time on task,
◆ communicates high expectations, and
◆ respects diverse talents and ways of learning.

Please note the conspicuous *absence* from this list of several time-
honored traditions in education: the extended lecture, the moral
exhortation (without skill building), the single bullet or method, and
the busywork (without impact or practicality).

As we transition in this chapter into presenting specific methods of EBP training, keep the broad evidence-based principles above
in mind and avoid resorting to discredited educational practices. In
other words, let us become evidence based about teaching EBPs.

Ensuring competence in EBPs requires explicit teaching and
evaluation of the requisite skills. Consider the task of teaching
complex psychotherapy skills to behavioral health and addiction
professionals. We'll use the example of motivational interviewing
(Miller & Rollnick, 2002), an evidence-based treatment for patients
such as Francesco, who deny or minimize their substance abuse.
The developers of motivational interviewing have systematically
evaluated their teaching methods. The least effective teaching
method involved doing nothing: a wait-list control group. Self-
guided training proved more effective than nothing. Attending a
clinical workshop proved superior to self-guided training, but participating in a workshop plus practice resulted in still better adoption. The most effective teaching method involved participating

in a workshop plus practice and coaching (Miller et al., 2004). Individual performance feedback and coaching improve the acquisition of clinical skills (Miller et al., 2006).

Interestingly, online training may prove just as effective as in-person workshops in promoting the use of EBPs. Several early studies (e.g., Dimeff et al., 2009; Rakovshik et al., 2016; Stein et al., 2015) demonstrated that with the same amount of training and follow-up supervision, online training led community clinicians to have as much knowledge and to adopt evidence-based treatments as much as traditional live trainings did. Internet-based training would enable many more practitioners to conveniently access EBP training. Note, however, that the studies mentioned did not simply provide online education but also involved personal supervision and consultation after the training.

These promising findings and online enhancements will probably converge into *blended learning* (or hybrid education) for implementing EBPs. **Blended learning** refers to the integration of multiple methods of information delivery into a single, coordinated learning system (Cucciare et al., 2008). Treatment manuals, training workshops, Web-based training, and subsequent supervision or consultation blend in ways that enhance learning, extend outreach, optimize practitioner time, and prove cost-effective. The supervision will probably need to remain in-person, even if it takes place at a distance via video chat, but EBP dissemination and training will increasingly experiment with novel delivery formats (Rotheram-Borus et al., 2012).

Learning multiple EBPs will prove more challenging than learning a single method because of the numerous skill sets required. Indeed, EBP involves both a conceptual framework and a skill set for clinical decision-making. In what follows, we offer teaching tips for explaining the EBP conceptual framework and imparting the EBP core skills. We also summarize nascent research on what clinicians prefer in their training in EBPs.

Conceptual Framework

The conceptual framework for EBP includes the professional expectation and individual commitment to incorporate the best available research into clinical practice. In our workshops, we fondly characterize our 15-minute talk on these central points as "Science is a candle in the dark" (Sagan, 1997). Any more than 15 minutes tends to generate student sighs, yawns, and eye-rolling. A compressed outline and sprinkling of examples from our pitch includes these points:

♦ Healthcare historically relied on nonresearch sources of information. In early days, practitioners followed theoretical doctrine, charismatic pioneers, subjective preferences, and clinical judgments. In modern days, practitioners increasingly look to empirical research to counter inevitable biases, clinical heuristics, and nonprobabilistic thinking.

♦ Controlled research remains incomplete and imperfect, of course, but superior to the alternatives. It represents our best, self-correcting method for making judicious and accurate decisions. The human mind tends to draw causality from coincidences; controlled research reliably tells us what works. We integrate recent examples from the mass media in which randomized clinical trial (RCT) results resolved ambiguity, for example, the controversies concerning hormone replacement therapy and the alleged curative value of magnets.

♦ Much of what we now practice derives from empirical research, largely but not exclusively RCTs. Compelling examples from behavioral health and the addictions include the superiority of actuarial judgment over clinical judgment in reaching diagnoses (Meehl, 1954), the comparability of outcomes obtained with psychoanalysis and briefer psychoanalytic psychotherapy (Wallerstein, 1986), the efficacy of teaching relapse prevention to addicted populations (Marlatt & Gordon, 1985), the inadvisability of using anatomically detailed dolls or puppets to determine whether or not a child experienced sexual abuse (Koocher et al., 1995), the centrality of the therapeutic relationship in predicting and contributing to successful psychotherapy outcomes (Norcross, 2011), and the ineffectiveness of various forms of confrontation in treating substance abuse (Miller et al., 2003).

♦ All of these robust research findings initially elicited reactions of "Impossible! Computers and statistical formulas will never outpredict the experienced human clinician—never!": Psychoanalysis obviously outperforms briefer therapies, which will obviously lead to symptom substitution and only fleeting improvement; relapse prevention will only "encourage relapse" rather than actually reduce the number of relapses. Many of today's standard clinical practices were initially branded as dubious, impossible, or heretical.

◆ Follow the guideposts of research when incorporating EBPs into clinical practice. Research informs us that collaborating with patients and reaching goal consensus lead to improved outcomes (Tryon & Winograd, 2011). Tailoring treatment to the individual patient, his or her preferences, and his or her characteristics also improves outcomes (Norcross, 2011). Research guides us in blending our clinical expertise with patient preferences. In fact, research has alerted us to those situations when clinical expertise might preempt the best available research. The EBP mantra of best available research, clinical expertise, and patient values derives directly and powerfully from the evidence!

◆ We should never consider EBP an academic exercise. On the contrary, it immediately helps you and your patients. Evidence-based practice improves outcomes for your individual patients as well as the health of the population. Effect sizes and probability values, we must remember, translate into vital human statistics: happier and healthier people.

Core Skills

As featured throughout the preceding chapters, the core EBP skills consist of formulating a specific, answerable clinical question (Chapter 2), accessing the best available research (Chapters 3 and 4), appraising that research evidence critically (Chapters 5–7), translating that research into practice with a particular patient (Chapter 8), integrating the clinician's expertise and patient's characteristics with the research (Chapter 9), and evaluating the effectiveness of the entire process (Chapter 10). Each of these core skills requires mastery by means of practice, coaching, and then implementation to insure they continue.

The research evidence (Bearman et al., 2013; Mazzucchelli & Sanders, 2010; NIRN, 2005) indicates that we can best teach each EBP skill by

◆ emphasizing practice of new skills;
◆ separating omnibus treatments into separate components or principles;
◆ using feedback on practice to teach the finer points;

- employing both positive and negative teaching examples;
- helping trainees integrate thinking and doing during practice sessions (didactic training tends to be linear, while practice tends to be multidimensional and dynamic);
- providing guidance with respect to the boundaries of using a particular skill or treatment, describing when it may be useful and when it may not;
- addressing cultural adaptations of the EBP (Whaley & Davis, 2007);
- requiring a minimal level of demonstrated competency in each skill;
- modeling and role playing more in supervision, as contrasted with discussion (more practice, less preaching); and
- encouraging flexible use of the method (within the bounds of fidelity).

In addition, clinical teachers of EBP (and EBM) have shared their favorite principles and strategies for helping students acquire the core skills (e.g., Wyer et al., 2004; Straus et al., 2005; Spring & Walker, 2007). Here's a sampling of their—and our—favorites:

- Dispute common myths about EBPs early so that students do not bring their contagious, learning-interfering resistances with them. Box 11.1 describes a dozen myths about EBPs in behavioral health and addictions.
- Make EBPs practical and immediate by using students' real-time cases; historical examples and the teacher's cases hold less relevance and fewer rewards for the learner.
- Capitalize on participants' natural curiosity and enthusiasm for helping: Once they realize that we do not expect them to calculate statistics or perform research, they are more likely to become highly engaged.
- Model EBPs in your own work. For example, when you encounter a difficult case, ask aloud about the underlying causes of the disorder, locate and appraise the research evidence, and discuss how the research does and does not apply to the specific patient.
- Teach to the learners' needs: Just as different patients require different strokes, your students will begin at different places, with disparate needs, motivations, and preferences.
- Work as an EBP team: Divide up the learning tasks and ask everyone to be responsible for a task.
- Use online tutorials to supplement instruction. Three exemplars for behavioral health and addictions are Evidence-Based Behavioral

---

Box 11.1 Twelve Myths about EBPs in Behavioral Health and Addictions

EBPs result in clinical work drained of individuality and creativity; they offer nothing but mindless cookbooks.

EBPs will stifle empathic, warm relationships; they ignore the patient–therapist relationship.

EBPs pertain only to cognitive–behavioral treatments in behavioral health; insight-oriented and relationship-based therapies are not and can never become EBPs.

EBPs represent financial rules to deprive practitioners of reimbursement and patients of services.

EBPs apply to doctoral-level, research-producing professionals, not direct-care practitioners.

EBPs ignore clinical expertise and patient preferences.

EBPs focus solely on knowledge gained from randomized clinical trials.

EBPs have arrived on the scene prematurely; we simply do not have sufficient research to guide us yet.

EBPs rarely if ever generalize to real-world patients; "my patients are different" from all those used in research studies.

EBPs will not catch on with senior clinicians; experienced practitioners do not alter their clinical behavior.

EBPs dismiss self-help groups such as Alcoholics Anonymous and other 12-step programs.

EBPs apply only to psychotherapy, not to assessment, prevention, diagnosis, and other critical decisions.

Adapted from Collins et al. (2007); Norcross et al. (2006a); Pagoto et al., 2007.

Practice at www.ebbp.org, the Centre for Evidence-Based Mental Health at www.cebmh.com, and the twelve online modules prepared in conjunction with this volume.

◆ Develop journal clubs around EBPs: Learn about advances that should change our practice and about how to handle vexing patient problems by using the best evidence.

◆ Teach with an eye toward lifelong learning: The goal should focus beyond practicing EBP a few times during training to inculcating a lifetime commitment.

♦ Orient clinic conferences, morning reports, and daily patient discussions around EBPs. To be sure, retain the typical sharing of clinical expertise about similar patients, but also strive to infuse these occasions with the best available research via literature searches, Cochrane Reviews, practice guidelines, and so on.

 Skill Exercise 11-3

Warning: This, the final skill exercise in this chapter and in this book, is the most ambitious one! Think of daily reports, weekly meetings, agency conferences, and other clinical gatherings in which you participate on a regular basis. Consider orienting one of them around EBPs—beginning with the research evidence and then adding clinician expertise and the patient contributions. Perhaps invite a healthcare librarian to show colleagues how to rapidly access the best available research and a local professor or researcher to weigh in. On occasion, invite clients to join the discussion to offer their unique consumer perspectives. Bring EBPs into routine practice.

This commitment to transfer of training, from initial training to daily practice, characterizes the most successful teaching of EBP. We seek both **maintenance**—consolidation and continuation of behavior change across time, usually after the training ends—and **generalization**—continuation of behavior change across patients and settings other than those included in training.

Fortunately, from educational and treatment research, we know a fair bit about how to accomplish maintenance and generalization (Kazdin, 2001). The following methods should become part of training programs from the beginning:

♦ Employ incentives for conducting EBP that the natural environment already provides.
♦ Involve the entire system of clinical and administrative staff; a single practitioner should not work as a lone EBP wolf.
♦ Gradually, not abruptly, fade out or discontinue the training program.

- Make the training situation as similar to the practice environment as possible.
- Begin with continuous and rich incentives for using EBPs, but then thin them out and delay them.
- Use peers and staff to facilitate continued use of EBPs.
- Assess and attend to slips back into previous, non-EBP behavior.
- Extend the length of training; brief training typically produces less maintenance and generalization.
- Add reminders and occasional booster training.

In all these ways, we can maintain the core EBP skills over time and generalize them to other clinical situations.

Mnemonics

Teachers and supervisors have developed mnemonics to provide easy and memorable ways for students to remember the EBP core skills. Some students (and teachers) appreciate these convenient tools for recalling the EBP steps, particularly in the early phase of training; others find them too cute or simplistic.

In EBM, the core skills are popularly known as the **five As**: *a*sk (a clinical question), *a*ccess (the research literature), *a*ppraise (the research), *a*pply (the research to a particular case), and *a*ssess (the effectiveness of the entire EBP process). In case conferences, clinical supervision, or staff meetings, practitioners routinely "work" the five As.

In behavioral health and addictions, the appraisal skill demands more detailed deliberations and more complicated decisions. For this reason, we have divided our treatment of this skill among three chapters (7, 8, and 9) and have concomitantly expanded the mnemonic. In our teaching and supervision, we use **AAA TIE** (or **triple A TIE**): *a*sk a specific clinical question, *a*ccess the research literature, *a*ppraise the research literature for its value, *t*ranslate the research into practice, *i*ntegrate the patient and the clinician with the research, and *e*valuate the entire process (including ethics).

4C/ID Model

One particular model has been successfully applied in higher and healthcare education to optimize the transfer of skills from the classroom to clinical practice: Four Component Instruction Design (4C/ID; van Merrienboer, 1997). As used in EBPs (Maggio et al., 2015), 4C/ID includes the four components of learning tasks, supportive information, procedural information, and part-task practice. Together, they guide a teaching process so as to avoid overloading the learner's cognitive abilities; integrate the knowledge, attitudes, and skills needed to execute a complex task; and increase transfer of skills to new situations.

Table 11.1 provides examples of potential learning tasks, supportive information, procedural information, and part-task practice for completing the AAA TIE for graduate students (working on a given case) and for practitioners (working with actual patients). Over several sessions, educators provide procedural and supportive knowledge and adopt the role of a coach on the part-task practice. Part tasks rapidly build to real-life, whole-task challenges, which facilitate the transfer of knowledge and skills to daily practice. We recommend that more healthcare educators embrace the 4C/ID model in designing and conducting EBP training in the classroom and the clinic (see Dolmans et al., 2013; Vandewaetere et al., 2015).

Clinician Preferences

What do clinicians want in and from EBPs? Recent studies have explored behavioral health clinicians' preferences for their training in EBPs (e.g., Herschell et al., 2014; Stewart & Chambless, 2009, 2010; Tasca et al., 2015; Wilson et al., 2009). The studies show generally consistent results that can directly inform teaching practices:

◆ Include several case examples, which render EBPs more compelling, as we love and learn from stories.
◆ Mention supportive research information, but tread lightly and summarize it.
◆ Involve supervisors, staff, and peers in the same training.
◆ Teach topics that are both relevant and appealing. (Disorders of leading interest seem to be post-traumatic stress disorder, depression, anxiety, and borderline personality disorder, while leading topics include the therapeutic relationship, mechanisms of change, therapist factors, professional development, and client factors.)

TABLE 11.1 Examples of EBP Training Activities Based on the Four Component Instructional Design (4C/ID) Model

Component	For graduate students	For practitioners
Learning tasks	Learners receive a written patient case (derived from real-life practice and focusing on a single, familiar condition) and a set of clinical questions, and are asked to complete the remaining EBP steps.	Learners identify a patient case from their own clinical experience and then identify a clinical question and execute all steps of EBP.
Supportive information	Learners read an article on appraising research critically and listen to a librarian describe her thought process for selecting databases.	Learners watch a short video of an experienced mental health practitioner thinking through her reasoning process aloud.
Procedural information	Learners receive a step-by-step handout to guide question formulation and are offered over-the-shoulder feedback from roving teachers while appraising research.	Learners are offered an online checklist to guide the critical appraisal of articles.
Part-task practice	Learners are provided with data on four screening tests and challenged to calculate the likelihood ratio for each test.	Learners do not engage in part-task practice if they have achieved mastery of the AAA TIE elements of EBP.

♦ Provide interactive training instead of using a lecture-based format.
♦ Consider the theoretical orientation of the participants, as cognitive–behavioral therapists tend to be more interested in

treatment of specific Axis I disorders, while psychodynamic therapists express more inclination toward Axis II (personality) disorders.

Implementing Evidence-Based Practices

Training practitioners effectively leads to initial acquisition of EBP skills but will not guarantee incorporation of EBPs into daily practice. Nor does training individual practitioners automatically yield EBP implementation throughout a unit or system of healthcare. But longer-term, multilevel implementation can maximize practitioners' behavior change and thus enhance healthcare outcomes.

That's the goal of **implementation science**: putting into routine practice an activity or program. It is an emerging, interdisciplinary field that investigates the methods that influence the integration of evidence-based interventions into practice settings and healthcare policy. By properly examining both individual behavior of practitioners and organizational systems of care, implementation scientists aim to reduce haphazard uptake of the research evidence.

The research consistently demonstrates that while EBP training improves practitioner knowledge of and attitude towards the EBP, long-term change in practitioner behavior occurs only when training is extensive and includes active learning (Beidas & Kendall, 2010). Here's what the research evidence—now totaling hundreds of individual studies—indicates will facilitate longer-term, multilevel implementation of EBPs (Fixsen et al., 2013; Greenhalgh et al., 2004; Mazzucchelli & Sanders, 2010; NIRN, 2005):

◆ Begin by conducting a readiness analysis of the system to identify factors likely to influence the proposed change.
◆ Secure the participation of local stakeholders and opinion leaders in the system or surrounding community.
◆ Collaborate with all the key stakeholders, including clinicians, consumers, family members, supervisors, insurance organizations, and mental health authorities; this process is known as **cocreation** in implementation science (Metz, 2015).
◆ Avoid single-bullet and time-limited interventions.
◆ Offer training to the entire staff (as described in the previous section).

◆ Provide training for trainers (and staff leaders) to maximize learning.
◆ Create peer support to build a culture of acceptance and support.
◆ Encourage the collection of clinical outcome data.
◆ Provide administrative and financial resources to sustain the changes.
◆ Build the PICO framework into record sheets, intake forms, and written documentation.
◆ Use patient-specific reminders at the point of care to prompt EBPs.
◆ Assess and track staff **fidelity** in using the EBPs.
◆ Monitor and evaluate the implementation.
◆ Reinforce and provide incentives for behavior changes toward EBPs.
◆ Insist that the new EBPs are conducted with fidelity before adapting them to local needs: "First do it right, then do it differently."
◆ Provide follow-up training and supervision to reduce practitioner drift.

The successful large-scale implementation of evidence-based treatments for children in the state of Hawaii provides a case in point (Chorpita et al., 2002). A multidisciplinary, academic-practice panel reviewed the vast literature on psychosocial treatments for childhood anxiety disorders, depression, ADHD, conduct disorders, and autistic disorder. The panel established a mental health system–university–parent partnership in working toward the design of practice guidelines. Subsequently, the state mental health system authorized a series of training workshops to provide practitioners with the skills to conduct the identified treatments and then revised a number of policies to support the continuing use of EBPs with children. All told, multiple stakeholders and multiple levels were involved in disseminating, teaching, and then implementing EBPs.

Consider as well the multiple structures and supports provided at three implementation levels (external, organizational, and individual) in Ohio. That state, like practically all states, has begun implementing behavioral health and substance abuse EBPs. Ohio worked at each level of influence to facilitate implementation of integrated dual-disorders treatment by state-contracted agencies and the state hospital system (Gotham, 2006). Externally, the state provided 2-year grants to nine treatment settings to insure implementation and support. Organizationally, the state provided consultation to the sites in the form of readiness assessments, implementation plans, site visits, fidelity self-studies, and outcomes monitoring. Individually, practitioners received a wide array of training, including statewide conferences, intensive on-site training, monthly follow-ups, and clinical supervision. That's precisely the type of longer-term, multi-level implementation that maximizes practitioners' behavior change and thus enhances healthcare outcomes.

Implementation of research-supported practices within healthcare systems occurs in predictable stages: exploration, adoption, program installation, initial implementation, full operation, innovation, and then sustainability (NIRN, 2005). **Sustainability** is achieved when the EBP becomes routinely executed with fidelity; that requires a functional infrastructure supporting the EBP for the long run. Reviews of leading implementation programs in behavioral health (e.g., Gallo & Barlow, 2012; McHugh & Barlow, 2012) find that sustainable programs regularly train the trainers, continue long-term consultation, establish peer consultation networks, and fund the EBPs in the agency's annual budget. There's a science to sustainability.

Think of systems implementation as a gradual process of behavior change, akin to a patient moving through the stages of change: pre-contemplation, contemplation, preparation, action, and maintenance (Prochaska et al., 1995, 2005). Each stage represents a period of time as well as a set of tasks needed for movement to the next stage. We need to consider an organization's readiness to change because each stage and each system will require something a little different.

The National Institute of Drug Abuse (NIDA) tries to do just that through its unique Clinical Trials Network (CTN), which partners treatment researchers with community-based practitioners in 19 geographic nodes throughout the United States (www.drugabuse.gov/about-nida/organization/cctn/ctn). The CTN first determines the effectiveness of a treatment for drug abuse across a broad range of community-based settings and diverse patient populations. Then it ensures the transfer and implementation of those research results to practitioners and patients. The core principle of the partnership is genuine bidirectionality between clinicians and researchers. Those involved in the regional CTN programs are more likely to adopt and use EBPs, and CTN has helped fuel the cultural shift toward evidence-based care for substance abusers and their families.

Thus, like EBP itself, implementation science sensitively integrates the best research evidence, clinical expertise, and staff characteristics and preferences into deciding what works for each unique healthcare system. That typically produces, as anticipated in Chapter 1, the overarching goals of EBP: more effective behavioral health services for our patients and enhanced public health for the populace.

Key Terms

AAA TIE (or triple A TIE)
blended learning
cocreation
dissemination
fidelity
five As

generalization
implementation
implementation science
maintenance
sustainability
translation(al) research

Recommended Readings and Websites

Addiction Technology Transfer Center Network, www.nattc.org/home/

Centre for Reviews and Dissemination (CRD), www.york.ac.uk/crd/

Institute of Behavioral Research. Organizational readiness for change, ibr.tcu.edu/publications/research-summaries/

McHugh, R. K., & Barlow, D. H. (Eds.). (2012). *Dissemination and implementation of evidence-based psychological interventions.* New York, NY: Oxford University Press.

Maggio, L. A., Cate, O., Irby, D. M., & O'Brien, B. C. (2015). Designing evidence-based medicine training to optimize the transfer of skills from the classroom to clinical practice: Applying the Four Component Instructional Design model. *Academic Medicine, 90,* 1457–1461.

Metz, A. (2015). *Implementation brief: The potential of co-creation in implementation science.* nirn.fpg.unc.edu/sites/nirn.fpg.unc.edu/files/resources/NIRN-Metz-ImplementationBreif-CoCreation.pdf

National Implementation Research Network (NIRN). Multiple documents, including the 2005 *Implementation research: A synthesis of the literature,* nirn.fpg.unc.edu/

NIDA Clinical Trials Network (CTN), www.drugabuse.gov/about-nida/organization/cctn/ctn

SAMHSA Evidence-Based Practice Toolkits, store.samhsa.gov/list/series?name=Evidence-Based-Practices-KITs

Spring, B., & Walker, B. B. (Eds.). (2007). Evidence-based practice in clinical psychology: Education and training issues [Special issue]. *Journal of Clinical Psychology, 63*(7).

Contents of Companion Website

URL: http://www.oup.com/us/cliniciansguide2e

Chapter	Topic
1	EBP Statements by Professional Organizations
3	Screenshots of Websites of Background and Filtered Sources
4	The Case of Juliette
4	Screenshots of Websites of Unfiltered Sources
5	Worksheet for Bonferroni Corrections
5	Websites for Power Calculations
5	Standard Errors of a Percentage and Confidence Intervals for p
5	Worksheet for Calculating Partial r
6	Conversion Formulas for Effect Sizes
9	Websites on Comorbid/Co-occurring Mental Health Disorders
10	Ethics Codes of Major Behavioral Health and Addiction Associations

Glossary

AAA TIE (or triple A TIE) In EBPs for mental health and addictions, a mnemonic for the core skills: *a*sk a specific clinical question; *a*ccess the research literature; *a*ppraise the research literature; *t*ranslate the research into practice; *i*ntegrate the patient and the clinician with the research; and *e*valuate the entire process, including ethics.

actuarial judgment Using numerical probabilities, as opposed to practitioner judgment, as a basis for clinical decisions; relies on empirically established statistical relationships between patient data and outcome.

adopt it, adapt it, or abandon it The three basic options for practitioners deciding how to proceed with a research-supported intervention in a particular case.

alpha level (α) A probability level (e.g., .05 or .01) used as a definition of a sufficiently low probability in a significance test that, if the obtained result falls below this level, the result is declared statistically significant.

analysis of covariance (ANCOVA) A type of analysis of variance that makes adjustments in the dependent variable used for comparing groups based on prior information about differences among the groups on some other variable.

analysis of variance (ANOVA) The technique(s) used to test the significance of main effects and interactions in a variety of research designs.

arbitrary metrics Psychological constructs rated with arbitrary numbers that tell us very little about the person in an absolute sense. For example, patients can rate their self-esteem as 5 out of 7 on a 7-point scale, and relative shifts in this rating can be tracked over time, but these scores cannot be meaningfully compared with another person's scores on the same test.

audit An examination of the performance of practitioners or service units, usually in terms of patient outcome in comparison to clinical standards, which might be general benchmarks, other practitioners, or EBP guidelines. The goal of an audit is to create an ongoing feedback loop to refine and improve the EBP evaluation process.

authority-based practice Basing clinical decisions and practices largely on the reputation and authority of a given healthcare practitioner; typically contrasted with **evidence-based practice**, which relies on solid research evidence.

background questions Broad clinical questions regarding general knowledge about disorders, tests, treatments, and other healthcare matters; they typically specify a question root (with a verb) followed by a disorder, treatment, or other healthcare issue. Contrast with **foreground questions.**

base rate The percentage of a population having a particular characteristic; often called the **prevalence rate** in the clinical literature.

benchmarks Comparative values that indicate desirable or "best practice" standards for assessing the effects of a service. In healthcare, benchmarking can address such matters as costs, staffing, waiting times, patient retention, and treatment outcomes.

best available research Clinically relevant research, often from basic health science, that will most likely yield accurate, unbiased, and relevant answers to a practice question posed for a particular patient or patient group. One of the three pillars of EBP.

blended learning The integration of multiple methods of information delivery into a single, coordinated learning system; also sometimes known as *hybrid instruction.*

BMJ Clinical Evidence A subscription resource for supporting clinical decision-making that summarizes evidence for over 2,000 treatments and preventative measures for more than 200 common health conditions.

Bonferroni correction A common method used to adjust the alpha level when more than one significance test is conducted within a single study. The correction involves dividing the nominal alpha level by the number of tests to be conducted.

Boolean operators Search commands used to logically connect search terms. The most common Boolean operators are AND, OR, and NOT.

Buros A common nickname for the *Mental Measurements Yearbook,* after its original editor, Oscar K. Buros.

Campbell Collaboration (C2) Shorthand for **Campbell Collaboration Reviews of Interventions and Policy Evaluations**.

Campbell Collaboration Reviews of Interventions and Policy Evaluations A database of over 120 systematic reviews focused on behavioral science evidence in the areas of education, social justice, and crime.

case study method A research design involving intensive observation and assessment of a single "case," be that a single individual, family, group, neighborhood, or community; typically lacks the controls and standardization of more rigorous research designs.

CINAHL The Cumulative Index to Nursing and Allied Health Literature, which provides access to citations for journal articles, books, chapters, dissertations, research instruments, and standards of practice.

clinical expertise Clinician skills that promote positive outcomes, including conducting assessments, developing diagnostic judgments, making clinical decisions, implementing treatments, monitoring patient progress, using interpersonal expertise, understanding cultural differences, and seeking available resources as needed. One of the three pillars of EBP.

Cochrane Shorthand for the Cochrane Database of Systematic Reviews.

Cochrane Database of Systematic Reviews (CDSR) A filtered database within the Cochrane Library comprising over 6,000 systematic reviews that synthesize available randomized clinical trials on a given healthcare topic.

cocreation Development of community partnerships and shared knowledge among important stakeholders to improve the acceptability, implementation, and sustainability of EBPs in the community.

Cohen's d A measure of effect size determined as the difference between two means divided by the pooled standard deviation for the two groups.

cohort A specified set of people with common characteristics followed over a specified period of time to determine the prevalence, etiology, complications, or prognosis (or some combination thereof) of a disorder.

comorbid disorders Two or more disorders occurring simultaneously.

confidence interval (CI) An interval around a statistic (e.g., a mean or correlation coefficient) within which the parameter estimated by the statistic should fall with a certain degree of probability, or an interval around an obtained test score within which the true score should fall with a certain degree of probability.

confirmatory factor analysis (CFA) A type of factor analysis that begins with a theory (model) about underlying dimensions in a set of measures and then tests how well the model fits; contrasted with exploratory factor analysis, which explores underlying dimensions without a prior theory.

confound A variable associated with or varying with an independent variable such that the effect of the independent variable cannot be separated from possible effects of the confound.

controlled vocabularies A curated list of terms that provides a standardized way of describing resources to facilitate the search and retrieval of information.

convenience samples Samples obtained by including cases simply because they are conveniently available; contrasted with probability samples.

core EBP skills In sequence, these practitioner competencies are asking a specific clinical question, accessing the best available research, appraising the research evidence critically, translating that research into practice with a particular patient, integrating the clinician's expertise and patient's characteristics with the research, and evaluating the effectiveness of the entire process. See also **AAA TIE.**

correction for attenuation A statistical correction applied to a correlation coefficient to account for imperfect reliability in one or both variables entering the correlation.

cost–benefit analysis A systematic way to estimate the strengths (benefits) and weaknesses (costs) of a proposed decision; the fundamental question involves whether the potential or likely beneficial outcomes outweigh the probable costs (e.g., time, expense, distress, side effects).

criterion problem The difficulty of determining what constitute appropriate criteria for determining effective treatment and who should decide on those criteria.

critical appraisal The process of assessing and interpreting research evidence by systematically considering its relevance to an individual's work.

cultural adaptation Modification of clinical services and programs in ways that are culturally sensitive and are tailored to a cultural group's worldviews.

cut score The score on a test that divides a group into discrete categories.

decision aids Written or electronic information that assists patients in selecting the best health treatment option for them by apprising them of the available treatments, identifying salient values, and describing the probable benefits and harms of each option.

decision analysis An approach for making decisions under conditions of uncertainty by modeling the sequences or pathways of possible strategies (e.g., diagnosis and treatment for a particular clinical problem). Its utility relies on estimates of the probabilities that particular events and outcomes will occur. Decision trees are often used to represent alternative pathways graphically (see Figures 8.1 and 8.2 for examples).

departure from standard of care A treatment course or behavior that many practitioners would not take. It raises a mild degree of liability risk should harm result, but it may seem reasonable to a percentage of practitioners if it possesses some documented effectiveness.

dependent variable In experimental design, the variable measured to determine if the independent variable had some effect. In correlational design, the variable predicted from the independent variable.

discredited practices Practices that are unable to consistently generate treatment outcomes (interventions) or valid data (assessments) beyond those obtained by the passage of time alone, expectancy, base rates, or credible placebos. The term *discredited* subsumes ineffective and detrimental interventions but forms a broader and more inclusive characterization.

dissemination The process of spreading and dispersing evidence-based materials to professionals and the public. See also **implementation**.

eMedicine A freely accessible evidence-based resource that provides background information for over 30 medical specialties.

effect size (ES) A measure of difference between means or a correlation coefficient indicating relative strength; it is calculated independently of measures of significance or random sampling fluctuations.

effect size benchmarks Selected levels indicating small, medium, and large effect sizes. Often referred to as *Cohen's benchmarks.*

effectiveness research A type of treatment study that shows the safety and outcomes of an intervention in real-world situations and that takes account of patient-, practitioner-, and system-level factors that may moderate the intervention's effect. Frequently contrasted with **efficacy research**.

efficacy research A type of treatment study employing well-controlled, time-limited conditions that maximize the likelihood of finding an intervention effect if one exists; the research findings do not necessarily transfer well to real-world situations. Frequently contrasted with **effectiveness research**.

epidemiology The study of how often and why diseases occur among different groups of people.

error score In classical test theory, the difference between a person's true score and obtained score; error is the result of unreliable variance.

ETS Test Collection An electronic, Web-accessible (www.ets.org/test_link/about) database providing basic, descriptive information for approximately 20,000 tests and measures.

evidence-based medicine (EBM) The integration of best available research evidence with clinical expertise and patient values. Closely related but not identical to **evidence-based practice**.

evidence-based practice (EBP) The integration of best available research with clinical expertise in the context of patient characteristics, culture, and preferences.

factor analysis A family of statistical techniques designed to identify dimensions (factors) accounting for the covariation in a multiplicity of variables.

false negatives In a 2 × 2 table showing the relationship between performance on a test and on an external criterion, cases that exceed the cut score on the criterion but not the cut score on the test.

false positives In a 2 × 2 table showing the relationship between performance on a test and on an external criterion, cases that exceed the cut score on the test but not the cut score on the criterion.

fidelity The degree to which an implemented practice adheres to the original treatment protocol; determining fidelity typically entails checking compliance with the EBP protocol and staff competence in conducting it.

filtered information sources Information sources that provide expert analysis and synthesis of individual studies and often make recommendations for practice.

five As A mnemonic for the five core skills in evidence-based medicine: *a*sk a clinical question, *a*ccess the research literature, *a*ppraise the research, *a*pply the research to a particular case, and *a*ssess the effectiveness.

foreground questions Specific clinical questions typically formatted in searchable PICO terms that include the patient, intervention, comparison, and outcome. Contrast with **background questions**.

four Ds of legal liability What a plaintiff must prove in a professional liability (malpractice) lawsuit: *d*ereliction of *d*uty that leads *d*irectly to *d*amages.

generalization A continuation of behavior change across real-life settings other than those included in treatment.

Google Scholar A multidisciplinary Web search engine for "scholarly sources" as identified by Google that includes journals, theses, books, institutional repositories, and conference proceedings.

gross negligence A treatment course or behavior that most practitioners would not take. When such behaviors lead to harm, significant liability accrues.

heuristics Mental operating procedures or "rules of thumb" that we usually apply unconsciously to help us perform abstract reasoning in cognitively economical ways. These strategies save us time and effort but typically fail when the data deviate from or fall outside our usual realms of expertise.

hits In a 2 × 2 table showing the relationship between performance on a test and on an external criterion, cases in which the test classification and the external criterion classification agree.

implementation The practical process of having practitioners actually use EBPs and thereby alter their clinical performance. See also **dissemination.**

implementation science The interdisciplinary field that investigates the methods that influence the integration of evidence-based interventions into practice settings and healthcare policy.

independent variable In experimental design, the variable being manipulated. In correlational design, the variable used to predict status on another variable.

interaction In a factorial design, the joint effect of two or more independent variables; a differential effect resulting from combinations of different levels of the independent variables.

logistic regression A set of techniques, similar to **multiple regression**, for expressing the degree of relationship between a dichotomous criterion variable and a composite of predictor variables, some of which may be discrete rather than continuous.

main effect In a factorial design, the direct effect of one of the independent variables on the dependent variable.

maintenance The consolidation and continuation of behavior change across time, usually after the treatment ends.

mediator The specific causal agent within a compound of elements that leads to changes in a dependent variable.

Medical Subject Headings The National Library of Medicine's subject heading system or controlled vocabulary that helps searchers generate targeted searches.

MEDLINE The premier database of the National Library of Medicine, currently containing over 25 million biomedical citations dating back to 1946. MEDLINE is the largest database within **PubMed**.

Mental Measurements Yearbook *(MMY)* A collection of professional reviews of tests. New editions appear approximately every three years; reviews are also available electronically.

meta-analysis A family of research techniques for formally combining or summarizing results from many studies of a given topic using the statistical results from the studies.

moderator A variable that interacts with an independent variable to influence outcomes on the dependent variable.

multiple regression A set of techniques to express the relationship between one variable (the criterion) and a composite of other variables, with the composite being constructed so as to apply optimal weights to each entry.

narrative review A summary of research studies on a single topic that depends on the review author's comprehension of the group of studies. Contrast with **meta-analysis.**

National Registry of Evidence-Based Programs and Practices (NREPP) A free filtered database of mental health and substance abuse programs with demonstrated efficacy.

natural language The language of everyday speech and use.

negative predictive power The percentage of cases that actually do not belong to a target group of all the cases falling below the **cut score** on a test.

null hypothesis The hypothesis that there is no difference between group means or no correlation between variables. Also sometimes called the *statistical hypothesis.* Contrast with **research hypothesis.**

null hypothesis significance test (NHST) The statistical mechanisms (e.g., *t*-test or *F*-test) for determining whether to accept or reject the **null hypothesis.**

obtained score In classical test theory, the score obtained by one individual on one occasion; also known as the *observed score.*

odds ratio (OR) The ratio between the rates of a particular characteristic in two groups, when rates are expressed as odds rather than base rates.

opportunistic bias The potential bias introduced by exploring data in multiple ways and then presenting the results in the most favorable, and publishable, manner.

OR confidence interval The **confidence interval** for an odds ratio; this confidence interval is asymmetrical around its OR.

outlier An aberrant or unusual data point; one that falls well outside the distribution of data points or the pattern(s) of relationship among variables.

paradoxical interventions Therapeutic techniques in which the clinician gives a patient (or family) an assignment that will probably be resisted but that will probably lead the patient to change in a desirable direction.

parameter A descriptive measure (e.g., mean or standard deviation) on a population; often estimated by its corresponding **statistic**.

partial correlation A procedure for expressing the degree of relationship between two variables with a third variable "held constant" or "partialed out."

patient characteristics, culture, and preferences The patient's personality, strengths, sociocultural context, unique concerns, and preferences brought to a clinical encounter that must be integrated into clinical decisions on how to best serve the patient. One of the three pillars of EBP.

(patient) preferences The behaviors or attributes of the treatment and practitioner that a patient values or desires. These form an essential part of the **patient characteristics, culture, and preferences** of EBP and a frequent means of adapting treatment to the individual.

pay for performance (P4P) A system of linking practitioner compensation to patient outcomes. Proposed models tend to recognize and reward clinicians whose aggregate outcome results show success relative to some agreed-upon measure (e.g., a pre- or postassessment, external benchmark, or criterion).

PICO Acronym for *patient, intervention, comparison,* and *outcome* used in formulating searchable clinical questions. Also known as *PICOT* when *type* of question is added.

placebo An action or substance administered to a group with the expectation that it will not have any meaningful effect; often administered to a control group contrasted with a treatment group.

positive predictive power The percentage of cases that actually belong to a target group of all the cases falling above the **cut score** on a test.

power In the context of statistical significance tests, the probability of *avoiding* **Type II error,** that is, the probability of rejecting the null hypothesis when it should be rejected because it is false. Power is defined as $1 - \beta$.

practice-based evidence An alternative or complement to **evidence-based practice** that favors collecting evidence of clinical effectiveness in real-world contexts, typically without true experimental designs; perceived by proponents as more accessible and culturally responsive than EBP.

practice guidelines Systematically developed statements designed to assist practitioner and patient decisions in specific clinical circumstances.

prevalence rate The percentage of a population having a particular characteristic; alternate name for **base rate.**

proportion of variance in common The degree of overlap or covariation between variables, especially as presented graphically in the form of overlapping geometric shapes or as a squared correlation (e.g., r^2, R^2).

PsycINFO A subscription database produced by the American Psychological Association that provides access to mental and behavioral health information, including over 4 million journal articles, books, and dissertations.

PsycTEST An electronic database with information about psychological tests, mostly unpublished, launched by the American Psychological Association in 2011; available by subscription only.

publication bias The tendency for research articles reporting new or statistically significant results to be published more frequently than articles reporting nonsignificant results; it complicates the interpretation of meta-analyses and systematic reviews.

PubMed A search engine for the biomedical literature operated by the National Library of Medicine that provides access to 25 million citations, including those indexed in **MEDLINE.**

random Having an equal probability of being selected or assigned to different groups or samples.

randomized clinical trial (RCT) The term used in clinical contexts to designate a **true experimental design**; also known as randomized controlled trial.

range restriction Restriction in the range or variance of scores, especially as such restriction affects the degree of correlation among variables.

relative risk The ratio between the rates for a particular characteristic in two groups, when rates are expressed as prevalences (base rates).

research hypothesis The hypothesis the researcher wishes to demonstrate or support. Also called the *scientific hypothesis*. Contrast with **null hypothesis.**

risk–benefit analysis A systematic way to quantify the ratio of potential risk to potential benefit to enable an informed decision.

risk management Retrospective evaluation for the prospective assessment of practice hazards. Risk management may involve addressing ethical violations, carelessness, simple errors, or even unfortunate outcomes without any actual negligence.

sensitivity The percentage of cases correctly identified by a test as being in the target group; also known as **selectivity.**

significance level Usually means the same as **alpha level.**

significance test The statistical test, usually of a null hypothesis and usually involving F, t, or χ^2, to determine if the **null hypothesis** should be rejected.

simple random sample A sample drawn from a population in such a way that each element of the population has an equal chance of being drawn into the sample.

specificity The percentage of cases correctly identified by a test as being in the nontarget group.

standard error of a statistic The standard deviation of a distribution of sample statistics around its parent population parameter. Used for statistical **significance tests** and **confidence intervals.**

standard error of measurement (*SEM*) The standard deviation of the distribution of many hypothetical obtained scores around the true score; an index of imprecision in the obtained score resulting from unreliable variance.

standard of care The prevailing professional judgment of peers engaged in similar activities to a practitioner in similar circumstances, given the knowledge the practitioner had or should have had at the time.

standardized mean difference The difference in means between two groups divided by some measure of group standard deviation; essentially the same as Cohen's *d*.

statistic A descriptive measure (e.g., mean or standard deviation) of a sample; often used to estimate a **parameter.**

statistical hypothesis See **null hypothesis.**

sustainability A stage of implementation in which an EBP is routinely executed with fidelity; typically requires a functional infrastructure that supports the EBP for the long run.

transdiagnostic Cutting across multiple diagnoses. Transdiagnostic research contrasts with research that includes only patients from a single diagnostic category.

translational research An inclusive term for the process of successfully moving research-supported discoveries into established healthcare practice and policy; includes **dissemination** and **implementation science**.

transportability The likelihood that an intervention found effective in one setting can be transported to a different setting with equal effectiveness.

treatment as usual (TAU) Treatment that patients would ordinarily receive in naturalistic healthcare settings, especially in contrast to a treatment under investigation.

TRIP An evidence-based search engine that delivers a combination of background, filtered, and unfiltered information.

triple A TIE See **AAA TIE**.

true experimental design A research design involving random assignment to groups, manipulation of an independent variable, and then measurement of a dependent variable comparing the groups. All variables other than the independent variable are controlled or allowed to vary at random among the groups.

true score In classical test theory, the score a person would receive on a perfectly reliable test; also conceptualized as the person's average score obtained after an infinite number of tests with varying forms, scorers, and occasions.

truncation A search tool that broadens a search by adding variations to the end of search terms, which can be helpful when searching for the plurals of search terms.

Type I error The probability of rejecting the null hypothesis when in fact it is true and should not be rejected. The probability of committing a Type I error is alpha (α). See also **alpha level.**

Type II error The probability of failing to reject the null hypothesis when in fact it is false and should be rejected. The probability of committing a Type II error is defined as beta (β).

unfiltered information sources Information sources that provide access to individual studies that need to be analyzed and synthesized.

UpToDate A topic overview resource, available by subscription, that is promoted as an evidence-based decision clinical support for point-of-care use that contains over 10,500 topic reviews from 23 specialties.

wild cards Search tools that broaden searches by automatically searching for variations of search terms; sometimes notated by the characters *, ?, $, and ! Wild cards can be applied to any part of a search term to signal the search system to identify alternate letters.

References

Aarons, G. A. (2006). Transformational and transactional leadership: Association with attitudes toward evidence-based practice. *Psychiatric Services, 57,* 1162–1169.

Aarons, G. A., Glisson, C., Hoagwood, K., Kelleher, K., Landsverk, J., & Cafri, G. (2010). Psychometric properties and U.S. national norms of the Evidence-Based Practice Attitude Scale (EBPAS). *Psychological Assessment, 22,* 356–365.

Addiction Technology Transfer Center Network, www.nattc.org/home/

Addis, M. E. (2002). Methods for disseminating research products and increasing evidence-based practice: Promises, obstacles, and future directions. *Clinical Psychology: Science and Practice, 9,* 367–378.

Alf, C., & Lohr, S. (2007). Sampling assumptions in introductory statistics classes. *American Statistician, 6,* 71–77.

American Psychological Association. (1994). *Diagnostic and statistical manual of mental disorders* (4th ed.). Washington, DC: Author.

American Psychological Association (2005). *Policy statement on evidence-based practice in psychology.* Washington, DC: Author.

American Psychological Association (2010a). *Ethical principles of psychologists and code of conduct.* Washington, DC: Author.

American Psychological Association (2010b). *Publication manual of the* American Psychological Association (6th ed.). Washington, DC: Author.

Anderson, N., Schlueter, J. E., Carlson, J. F., & Geisinger, K. F. (Eds.). (2016). *Tests in print IX.* Lincoln, NE: Buros Center for Testing.

Anderson, S. A., & Maxwell, S. E. (2016). There's more than one way to conduct a replication study: Beyond statistical significance. *Psychological Methods, 21*(1), 1–12.

APA Task Force on Evidence-Based Practice. (2006). Evidence-based practice in psychology. *American Psychologist, 61,* 271–285.

Bachman, J. (2006). Pay for performance in primary and specialty behavioral health care: Two "concept" proposals. *Professional Psychology: Research and Practice, 37*(4), 384–388.

Barkham, M., Hardy, G. E., & Mellor-Clark, J. (Eds.) (2010). *Developing and delivering practice-based evidence: A guide for the psychological therapies.* Chichester, UK: Wiley.

Baugh, F. (2001). Correcting effect sizes for score reliability. *Educational and Psychological Measurement, 62,* 254–263.

Bearman, S. K., Weisz, J. R., Chorpita, B. F., Hoagwood, K., Ward, A., Ugeto, A. M., & Bernstein, A. (2013). More practice, less preach? The role of supervision processes and therapist characteristics in EBP implementation. *Administration and Policy in Mental Health Services, 40,* 518–529.

Begley, S. (2007, May 7). Just say no—to bad science. *Newsweek,* 57.

Beidas, R. S., & Kendall, P. C. (2010). Training therapists in evidence-based practice: A critical review of studies from a systems-contextual perspective. *Clinical Psychology: Science and Practice, 17,* 1–30.

Bennett, B. E., Bricklin, P. M., Harris, E. A., Knapp, S., VandeCreek, L., & Youngreen, J. N. (2007). *Assessing and managing risk in psychological practice: An individualized approach.* Rockville, MD: American Psychological Association Insurance Trust.

Berke, D. M., Rozell, C. A., Hogan, T. P., Norcross. J. C., & Karpiak, C. P. (2011). What clinical psychologists know about evidence-based practice: Familiarity with online resources and research methods. *Journal of Clinical Psychology, 67,* 1–11.

Bernal, G., & Domenech Rodriguez, M. M. (Eds.). (2012). *Cultural adaptations: Tools for evidence-based practice with diverse populations*. Washington, DC: American Psychological Association.

Beutler, L. E., Harwood, T. M., Kimpara, S., Verdirame, D., & Blau, K. (2011a). Coping style. In J. C. Norcross (Ed.), *Psychotherapy relationships that work* (2nd ed., pp. 336–353). New York, NY: Oxford University Press.

Beutler, L. E., Harwood, T. M., Michelson, A., Song, X., & Holman, J. (2011b). Reactance/resistance. In J. C. Norcross (Ed.), *Psychotherapy relationships that work* (2nd ed., pp. 261–278). New York, NY: Oxford University Press.

Bjorstad, G., & Montgomery, P. (2005). Family therapy for attention-deficit disorder or attention-deficit/hyperactivity disorder in children and adolescents. Cochrane Database of Systematic Reviews, www.cochrane.org/reviews/en/ab005042.html

Blanton, H., & Jaccard, J. (2006). Arbitrary metrics in psychology. *American Psychologist, 61*(1), 27–41.

BMC Medical Informatics and Decision Making, www.biomedcentral.com/bmcmedinformdecismak

Bohart, A. C. (2005). The active client. In J. C. Norcross, L. E. Beutler, & R. F. Levant (Eds.), *Evidence-based practices in mental health: Debate and dialogue on the fundamental questions*. Washington, DC: American Psychological Association.

Bohart, A., & Tallman, K. (1999). *How clients make therapy work: The process of active self-healing*. Washington DC: American Psychological Association.

Borenstein, M., Hedges, L. V., Higgins, J. P. T., & Rothstein, H. R. (2009). *Introduction to meta-analysis*. Hoboken, NJ: Wiley.

Bowden-Jones, O., Iqbal, M. Z., Tyrer, P., Seivewright, N., Cooper, S., Judd, A., & Weaver, T. (2004). Prevalence of personality disorder in alcohol and drug services and associated comorbidity. *Addiction, 99*, 1306–1314.

Brennan, R. L. (2001). *Generalizability theory*. New York, NY: Springer.

Brown, T. A. (2015). *Confirmatory factor analysis for applied research* (2nd ed.). New York, NY: Guilford.

Cabral, R. R., & Smith, T. B. (2011). Racial/ethnic matching of clients and therapists in mental health services: A meta-analytic review of preferences, perceptions, and outcomes. *Journal of Counseling Psychology, 58,* 537–554.

Calculating risks of harm, www.clinicalevidence.com/ceweb/resources/calculate_risk.jsp

Carlson, J. F., Geisinger, K. F., & Jonson, J. L. (Eds.). (2017). *The twentieth mental measurements yearbook.* Lincoln, NE: Buros Center for Testing.

Castonguay, L. G., & Beutler, L. E. (Eds.). (2005). *Principles of Therapeutic Change that Work.* New York, NY: Oxford University Press.

Castro, F. G., Barrera, M., & Martinez, C. R. (2004). The cultural adaptation of prevention interventions: Resolving tensions between fit and fidelity. *Prevention Science, 5,* 41–45.

Centre for Evidence-Based Medicine, www.cebm.net

Centre for Evidence-Based Medicine. Applying evidence to patients. ktclearinghouse.ca/cebm/practise/apply

Centre for Evidence-Based Mental Health, www.cebmh.com

Centre for Health Evidence, www.cche.net

Centre for Reviews and Dissemination (CRD), www.york.ac.uk/crd/

Chambless, D. L., & Crits-Christoph, P. (2005). The treatment method. In J. C. Norcross, L. E. Beutler, & R. F. Levant (Eds.), *Evidence-based practices in mental health: Debate and dialogue on the fundamental questions.* Washington, DC: American Psychological Association.

Chickering, A. W., & Gamson, Z. F. (1987, March). Seven principles for good practice in undergraduate education. *AAHE Bulletin,* 3–7.

Chorpita, B. F., Yim, L. M., Donkervoet, J. C., Arensdorf, A., Amundsen, M. J., McGee, C., . . . Morelli, P. (2002). Toward large-scale implementation of empirically supported treatments for children: A review and observations by the Hawaii Empirical Basis to Services Task Force. *Clinical Psychology: Science and Practice, 9,* 165–190.

Coburn, K. M., & Vevea, J. L. (2015). Publication bias as a function of study characteristics. *Psychological Methods, 20*(3), 310–330.

Cochrane, A. L. (1979). 1931–1971: A critical review with particular reference to the medical profession. In *Medicines for the year 2000* (pp. 1–11). London, UK: Office of Health Economics.

Cohen, J. (1988). *Statistical power analysis for the behavioral sciences* (2nd ed.). Hillsdale, NJ: Erlbaum.

Cohen, J., Cohen, P., West, S. G., & Aiken, L. S. (2003). *Applied multiple regression/correlation analysis for the behavioral sciences* (3rd ed.). Mahwah, NJ: Erlbaum.

Collins, F. L., Leffingwell, T. R., & Belar, C. D. (2007). Teaching evidence-based practice: Implications for psychology. *Journal of Clinical Psychology, 63,* 657–670.

Cone, J. D. (2000). *Evaluating outcomes: Empirical tools for effective practice.* Washington, DC: American Psychological Association.

CONSORT, www.consort-statement.org/

Cucciare, M. A., Weingardt, K. R., & Villafranca, S. (2008). Using blended learning to implement evidence-based psychotherapies. *Clinical Psychology: Science and Practice, 15,* 299–307.

Cumming, G. (2012). *Understanding the new statistics: Effect sizes, confidence intervals, and meta-analysis.* New York, NY: Routledge.

Daubert v. Merrell Dow Pharmaceuticals, Inc., 509 U.S. 579, 113 S. Ct. 2786 (1993).

DeCoster, J., Sparks, E. A., Sparks, J. C., Sparks, G. G., & Sparks, C. W. (2015). Opportunistic biases: Their origins, effects, and an integrated solution. *American Psychologist, 70,* 499–514. doi:10.1037/a0039191

Del Fiol, G., Workman, T. E., & Gorman, P. N. (2014). Clinical questions raised by clinicians at the point of care: A systematic review. *JAMA Internal Medicine, 174*(5), 710–718.

De Los Reyes, A., & Kazdin, A. E. (2004). Measuring informant discrepancies in clinical child research. *Psychological Assessment, 16,* 330–334.

De Los Reyes, A., & Kazdin, A. E. (2008). When the evidence says, "Yes, no, and maybe so." Attending to and interpreting inconsistent findings among evidence-based interventions. *Current Directions in Psychological Science, 17,* 47–51.

DiClemente, C. C. (2006). *Addiction and change: How addictions develop and addicted people recover.* New York, NY: Guilford.

Dimeff, L. A., Koerner, K., Woodcock, E. A., Beadnell, B., Brown, M. Z., Skutch, J. M., . . . Harned, M. S. (2009). Which training method works best? A randomized controlled trial comparing three methods of training clinicians in dialectical behavior therapy. *Behavior Research and Therapy, 47,* 921–930.

Division of Biostatistics, Department of Epidemiology and Biostatistics, School of Medicine, University of California, San Francisco (2006). Power and sample size programs [Computer software]. www.biostat.ucsf.edu/sampsize.html

Dolmans, D. H., Wolfhagen, I. H., & Van Merriënboer, J. J. (2013). Twelve tips for implementing whole-task curricula: How to make it work. *Medical Teacher, 35,* 801–805.

ETS Test Collection, www.ets.org/test_link/about

Evidence-Based Behavioral Practice, www.ebbp.org

Evidence-Based Practice for the Helping Professions, www.evidence. brookscole.com

Farmer, R. F., & Chapman, A. L. (2016). *Behavioral interventions in cognitive behavior therapy: Practical guidance for putting theory into action.* Washington, DC: American Psychological Association.

Farnsworth, J., Hess, J., & Lambert, M. J. (2001, April). *A review of outcome measurement practices in the* Journal of Consulting and Clinical Psychology. Paper presented at the annual meeting of the Rocky Mountain Psychological Association, Reno, NV.

Figueira, J., Greco, S., & Ehrgott, M. (Eds.). (2005). *Multiple criteria decision analysis: State of the art surveys.* New York, NY: Springer.

Fixsen, D., Blasé, K., Metz, A., & Van Dyke, M. (2013). Statewide implementation of evidence-based programs. *Exceptional Children, 79,* 213–230.

Formulating Answerable Clinical Questions, ktclearinghouse.ca/cebm/practise/formulate/

Gallo, K. P., & Barlow, D. H. (2012). Factors involved in clinician adoption and nonadoption of evidence-based interventions in mental health. *Clinical Psychology: Science and Practice, 19,* 93–106.

Gambrill, E. (2012). *Critical thinking in clinical practice: Improving the quality of judgments and decisions* (3rd ed.). Hoboken, NJ: Wiley.

Garb, H. N. (1998). Clinical judgment. In H. N. Garb (Ed.), *Studying the clinician: Judgment research and psychological assessment* (pp. 173–206). Washington, DC: American Psychological Association.

Garson, G. D. (2013). *Survey research and sampling.* Asheboro, NC: Statistical Publishing Associates.

Geisinger, K. F., Spies, R. A., Carlson, J. F., & Plake, B. S. (2007). *The seventeenth mental measurements yearbook.* Lincoln: University of Nebraska Press.

Gilovich, T., Griffin, D., & Kahneman, D. (Eds.). (2002). *Heuristics and biases: The psychology of intuitive judgment.* New York, NY: Cambridge University Press.

Giustini, D., & Barsky, E. (2005). A look at Google Scholar, PubMed, and Scirus: Comparisons and recommendations. *Journal of the Canadian Health Libraries Association, 26*(3), 85.

Gotham, H. J. (2004). Diffusion of mental health and substance abuse treatments: Development, dissemination, and implementation. *Clinical Psychology: Science and Practice, 11,* 160–176.

Gotham, H. J. (2006). Advancing the implementation of evidence-based practices into clinical practice: How do we get there from here? *Professional Psychology: Research and Practice, 37,* 606–613.

Greene, B., Bieschke, K. J., Perez, R. M., & DeBord, K. A. (2007). Delivering ethical psychological services to lesbian, gay, and bisexual clients. In R. M. Perez, K. A. DeBord, & K. J. Bieschke (Eds.), *Handbook of counseling and psychotherapy with lesbian, gay, bisexual, and transgender clients* (2nd ed., pp. 181–199). Washington, DC: American Psychological Association.

Greenhalgh, T., Robert, G. Macfarlane, F., Bate, P., & Kyriakidou, O. (2004). Diffusion of innovations in service organizations: Systematic review and recommendations. *Milbank Qurterly, 82,* 581–629.

Greer, A. (1994). Scientific knowledge and social consensus. *Controlled Clinical Trials, 15,* 431–436.

Grissom, R. J., & Kim, J. J. (2012). *Effect sizes for research: Univariate and multivariate applications* (2nd ed.). New York, NY: Taylor & Francis.

Guyatt, G., & Rennie, D. (Eds.). (2002). *Users' guides to the medical literature: Essentials of evidence-based clinical practice.* Chicago, IL: American Medical Association.

Guyatt, G., Rennie, D., Meade, M. O., & Cook, D. J. (2008). *Users' guides to the medical literature: Essentials of evidence-based clinical practice* (2nd ed.). Chicago, IL: McGraw-Hill.

Hannan, C., Lambert, M. J., Harmon, C., Nielsen, S. L., Smart, D. W., Shimokawa, K., & Sutton, S. W. (2005). A lab test and algorithms for identifying clients at risk for treatment failure. *Journal of Clinical Psychology: In Session, 61,* 155–163.

Hayes, A. F. (2013). *Introduction to mediation, moderation, and conditional process analysis: A regression-based approach.* New York, NY: Guilford.

Herschell, A. D., Reed, A. J., Mecca, L. P., & Kolko, D. J. (2014). Community-based clinicians' preferences for training in evidence-based practices: A mixed-method study. *Professional Psychology: Research and Practice, 45*, 188–199.

Hoagwood, K. (2002). Making the translation from research to its application: The *je ne sais pas* of evidence-based practices. *Clinical Psychology: Science and Practice, 9*, 210–213.

Hogan, T. P. (2005). Sources of information about psychological tests. In G. P. Koocher, J. C. Norcross, & S. S. Hill (Eds.), *Psychologist's desk reference* (2nd ed., pp. 105–107). New York, NY: Oxford University Press.

Hogan, T. P., & Evalenko, K. (2006). The elusive definition of outliers in introductory statistics textbooks. *Teaching of Psychology, 33*, 252–256.

Holahan, C. J., Moos, R. H., Holahan, C. K., Brennan, P. L., & Schutte, K. K. (2005). Stress generation, avoidance coping, and depressive symptoms: A 10-year model. *Journal of Consulting and Clinical Psychology, 73*, 658–666.

Hosmer, D. W., Jr., Lemeshow, S., & Sturdivant, R. X. (2013). *Applied logistic regression* (3rd ed.). Hoboken, NJ: Wiley.

How to use the Cochrane Library, www.cochranelibrary.com/help/how-to-use-cochrane-library.html

Huang, X., Lin, J., & Demmer-Fushman, D. (2006, November). *PICO as knowledge representation for clinical questions.* Paper presented at the annual symposium of the American Medical Informatics Association, Washington, DC. Available from www.umiacs.umd.edu/~jimmylin/publications/Huang-etal-AMIA2006.pdf

Hunink, M. G. M., Weinstein, M. C., Wittenberg, E., Drummond, M. F., Pliskin, J. S., Wong, J. B., & Glasziou, P. P. (2014). *Decision making in health and medicine: Integrating evidence and values* (2nd ed.). Cambridge, UK: Cambridge University Press.

Hunsley, J., Crabb, R., & Mash, E. J. (2004). Evidence-based clinical assessment. *The Clinical Psychologist, 57*(3), 25–32.

Hunsley, J., & Lee, C. M. (2007). Research-informed benchmarks for psychological treatments: Efficacy studies, effectiveness studies, and beyond. *Professional Psychology: Research and Practice, 38*, 21–33.

Hunsley, J., & Mash, E. J. (Eds.). (2008). *A guide to assessments that work.* New York, NY: Oxford University Press.

Hunter, J. E., & Schmidt, F. L. (2015). *Methods of meta-analysis: Correcting error and bias in research findings* (3rd ed.). Thousand Oaks, CA: Sage.

Institute of Behavioral Research. Organizational readiness for change, ibr.tcu.edu/publications/research-summaries/

Institute of Medicine (2001). *Crossing the quality chasm: A new health system for the 21st century.* Washington, DC: National Academies Press.

Isaacs, D., & Fitzgerald, D. (1999). Seven alternatives to evidence based medicine. *British Medical Journal, 319,* 1618.

Jacobson, R. (2015, October 21). Many antidepressant studies found tainted by pharma company influence. *Scientific American.* www.scientificamerican.com/article/many-antidepressant-studies-found-tainted-by-pharma-company-influence/

Jensen-Doss, A., Hawley, K. M., Lopez, M., & Osterberg, L. D. (2009). Using evidence-based treatments: The experience of youth providers working under a mandate. *Professional Psychology: Research and Practice, 40,* 417–424.

Jette, D. U., Bacon, K., Batty, C., Carlson, M., Ferland, A., Hemingway, R. D., . . . Volk, D. (2003). Evidence-based practice: Beliefs, attitudes, knowledge, and behaviors of physical therapists. *Physical Therapy, 93,* 78–96.

Kahneman, D., & Tversky, A. (Eds.). (2000). *Choices, values, and frames.* New York, NY: Cambridge University Press.

Karpiak, C. P., & Zaboski, B. A. (2013). Lifetime prevalence of mental disorders in the general population. In G. P. Koocher, J. C. Norcross, & B. A. Greene (Eds.), *Psychologists' desk reference* (3rd ed., pp. 3–16). New York, NY: Oxford.

Kazdin, A. (2001). *Behavior modification in applied settings* (6th ed.). Belmont, CA: Thomson Wadsworth.

Kazdin, A. E. (2005). *Parent management training.* New York, NY: Oxford University Press.

Kazdin, A. E. (2006). Arbitrary metrics: Implications for identifying evidence-based treatments. *American Psychologist, 61*(1), 42–49.

Kennedy, J. J. (1992). *Analyzing qualitative data: Log-linear analysis for behavioral research* (2nd ed.). New York, NY: Praeger.

Kenny, D. A. (2015). Mediate [Website on mediation analysis]. davidakenny.net/dtt/mediate.htm

Kent, D., & Hayward, R. (2007). When averages hide individual differences in clinical trials. *American Scientist, 95,* 60–72.

Kessler, R. C., Chiu, W. T., Demler, O., & Walters, E. E. (2005). Prevalence, severity, and comorbidity of 12-month DSM-IV disorders in the National Comorbidity Survey Replication. *Archives of General Psychiatry, 62,* 617–627.

Kirk, R. E. (2013). *Experimental design: Procedures for the behavioral sciences* (4th ed.). Thousand Oaks, CA: Sage.

Klimes-Dougan, B., August, G. J., Lee, C. Y. S., Realmuto, G. M., Bloomquist, M. L., Horowitz, J. L., & Eisenberg, T. L. (2009). Practitioner and site characteristics that relate to fidelity of implementation: The Early Risers prevention program in a going-to-scale intervention trial. *Professional Psychology: Research and Practice, 40,* 467–475.

Kline, R. B. (2011). *Principles and practice of structural equation modeling* (3rd ed.). New York, NY: Guilford.

Knapp, S., Younggren, J. N., VandeCreek, L., Harris, E., and Martin, J. N. (2013). Assessing and managing risk in psychological practice: An individualized approach (2nd ed.). Bethesda, MD: The Trust.

Knollmann, B. C. (Ed.). (2011). *Goodman & Gilman's The pharmacological basis of therapeutics* (12th ed.). New York, NY: McGraw-Hill Medical.

Koocher, G. P., Goodman, G. S., White, S., Friedrich, W. N., Sivan, A. B., & Reynolds, C. R. (1995). Psychological science and the use of anatomically detailed dolls in child sexual abuse assessments. *Psychological Bulletin, 118,* 199–222.

Koocher, G. P., & Keith-Spiegel, P. (2016). *Ethical principles in psychology and the mental health professions: Standards and cases* (4th ed.). New York, NY: Oxford University Press.

Koocher, G. P., McMann, M. R., Stout, A. O., & Norcross, J. C. (2014). Discredited assessment and treatment methods used with children and adolescents: A Delphi poll. *Journal of Clinical Child and Adolescent Psychology, 44,* 722–729.

Kruger, J., & Dunning, D. (1999). Unskilled and unaware of it: How difficulties in recognizing one's own incompetence lead to inflated self-assessments. *Journal of Personality Assessment and Social Psychology, 77,* 1121–1134.

Kumho Tire Co., Ltd. v. Carmichael, 119 S. Ct. 1167 (1999).

Lambert, M. J. (2010). *Prevention of treatment failure: The use of measuring, monitoring, and feedback in clinical practice.* Washington, DC: American Psychological Association.

Lambert, M. J. (Ed.). (2013). *Bergin and Garfield's handbook of psychotherapy and behavior change* (6th ed). New York, NY: Wiley.

Lambert, M. J., & Ogles, B. M. (2004). The efficacy and effectiveness of psychotherapy. In M. J. Lambert (Ed.), *Bergin and Garfield's handbook of psychotherapy and behavior change* (4th ed., pp. 139–193). New York, NY: Wiley.

Lau, A. S. (2006). Making the case for selective and directed cultural adaptations of evidence-based treatments: Examples from parent training. *Clinical Psychology: Science and Practice, 13*, 295–310.

Lewczy, C. M., Garland, A. F., Hurlburt, M. S., Gerrity, J., & Hough, R. L. (2003). Comparing DISC-IV and clinician diagnoses among youths receiving mental health services. *Journal of the American Academy of Child and Adolescent Psychiatry, 42*, 349–356.

Lilienfeld, S. O. (2007). Psychological treatments that cause harm. *Perspectives on Psychological Science, 2*, 53–70.

Luborsky, L., Diguer, L., Seligman, D. A., Rosenthal, R., Krause, E. D., Johnson, S., . . . Schweizer, E. (1999). The researcher's own therapy allegiances: A "wild card" in comparisons of treatment efficacy. *Clinical Psychology: Science and Practice, 6*, 95–106.

Lundh, A., Sismondo, S., Lexchin, J., Busuioc, O. A., & Bero, L. (2012). Industry sponsorship and research outcome. *Cochrane Library.* doi:10.1002/14651858.MR000033.pub2

Maggio, L. A., Cate, O., Irby, D. M., & O'Brien, B. C. (2015). Designing evidence-based medicine training to optimize the transfer of skills from the classroom to clinical practice: Applying the Four Component Instructional Design model. *Academic Medicine, 90*, 1457–1461.

Maggio, L. A., Tannery, N. H., & Kanter, S. L. (2011). AM last page: How to perform an effective database search. *Academic Medicine, 86*(8), 1057.

Magnavita, J. J. (Ed.). (2016). Clinical decision-making in mental health practice. Washington, DC: American Psychological Association.

Marlatt, G. A., & Gordon, J. R. (Eds.). (1985). *Relapse prevention: Maintenance strategies in addictive behavior change.* New York, NY: Guilford.

Mazzucchelli, T. G., & Sanders, M. R. (2010). Facilitating practitioner flexibility within an empirically supported intervention: Lessons for a system of parenting support. *Clinical Psychology: Science and Practice, 17*, 238–252.

McGlashan, T. H., Grilo, C. M., Skodol, A. E., Gunderson, J. G., Shea, M. T., Morey, L. C., . . . Stout, R. L. (2000). The Collaborative Longitudinal Personality Disorders Study: Baseline Axis I/II and II/II diagnostic co-occurrence. *Acta Psychiatrica Scandinavica, 102,* 256–264.

McHugh, R. K., & Barlow, D. H. (Eds.). (2012). *Dissemination and implementation of evidence-based psychological interventions.* New York, NY: Oxford University Press.

Meehl, P. E. (1954). *Clinical vs. statistical prediction.* Minneapolis: University of Minnesota Press.

Mentz, R. J., Hernandez, A. F., Berdan, L. G., Rorick, T., O'Brien, E. C., Ibarra, J. C., . . . Peterson, E. D. (2016). Good clinical practice guidance and pragmatic clinical trials: Balancing the best of both worlds. *Circulation, 133*(9), 872–880.

Mesgari, M., Okoli, C., Mehdi, M., Nielsen, F. Å., & Lanamäki, A. (2015). "The sum of all human knowledge": A systematic review of scholarly research on the content of Wikipedia. *Journal of the Association for Information Science and Technology, 66,* 219–245.

Messer, S. B. (2004). Evidence-based practice: Beyond empirically supported treatments. *Professional Psychology: Research and Practice, 36,* 580–588.

Metz, A. (2015). *Implementation brief: The potential of co-creation in implementation science.* nirn.fpg.unc.edu/sites/nirn.fpg.unc.edu/files/resources/NIRN-Metz-ImplementationBreif-CoCreation.pdf

Michels, R. (1984). *Differential therapeutics in psychiatry.* New York, NY: Brunner/Mazel.

Miller, P. M., & Kavanagh, D. J. (Eds.). (2007). *Translation of addictions science into practice.* London, UK: Elsevier.

Miller, S. D., Duncan, B. L., Sorrell, R., & Brown, G. S. (2005). The Partners for Change outcome management system. *Journal of Clinical Psychology: In Session, 61,* 199–208.

Miller, W. R., & Rollnick, S. (2002). *Motivational interviewing: Preparing people for change.* New York, NY: Guilford.

Miller, W. R., Sorensen, J. L., Selzer, J. A., & Brigham, G. S. (2006). Disseminating evidence-based practices in substance abuse treatment: A review with suggestions. *Journal of Substance Abuse Treatment, 31,* 25–39.

Miller, W. R., Wilbourne, P. L., & Hettema, J. E. (2003). What works? A summary of alcohol treatment outcome research. In R. K.

Hester & W. R. Miller (Eds.), *Handbook of alcoholism treatment approaches* (3rd ed., pp. 13–63). Boston, MA: Allyn & Bacon.

Miller, W. R., Yahne, C. E., Moyers, T. B., Martinez, J., & Pirritano, M. (2004). A randomized trial of methods to help clinicians learn motivational interviewing. *Journal of Consulting and Clinical Psychology, 72,* 1050–1062.

Moffitt, T. E., Harrington, H. L., Caspi, A., Kim-Cohen, J., Goldberg, D., Gregory, A. M., & Poulton, R. (2007). Depression and generalized anxiety disorder: Cumulative and sequential comorbidity in a birth cohort followed prospectively to age 32 years. *Archives of General Psychiatry, 64,* 651–660.

Moher, D., Schulz, K. F., & Altman, D. G. (2001a). CONSORT e-checklist and flowchart. www.consort-statement.org/downloads

Moher, D., Schulz, K. F., & Altman, D. G. (2001b). The CONSORT statement: Revised recommendations for improving the quality of reports of parallel-group randomized trials. *Annals of Internal Medicine, 134,* 657–662.

Nathan, P. E., & Gorman, J. M. (Eds.). (2015). *A guide to treatments that work* (4th ed.). New York, NY: Oxford University Press.

National Advisory Mental Health Council on Behavioral Science (2000). *Translating behavioral science into action: Report of the National Advisory Mental Health Council's Behavioral Science Workgroup* (No. 00-4699). Bethesda, MD: National Institute of Mental Health.

National Comorbidity Survey Replication. (2005). *National Comorbidity Survey (NCS) and National Comorbidity Survey Replication (NCS-R).* www.hcp.med.harvard.edu/ncs/

National Guideline Clearinghouse, www.guideline.gov

National Implementation Research Network (NIRN). (2005). *Implementation research: A synthesis of the literature.* nirn.fpg.unc.edu/sites/nirn.fpg.unc.edu/files/resources/NIRN-MonographFull-01-2005.pdf

National Institute for Health and Clinical Excellence, www.nice.org.uk

National Registry of Evidence-Based Programs and Practices, www.nrepp.samhsa.gov

Nelson, T. D., & Steele, R. G. (2007). Predictors of practitioner self-reported use of evidence-based practices: Practitioner training, clinical setting, and attitudes toward research. *Administration and Policy in Mental Health, 34*(4), 319–330.

NIDA Clinical Trials Network (CTN), www.drugabuse.gov/about-nida/organization/cctn/ctn

Norcross, J. C. (Ed.). (2011). *Psychotherapy relationships that work* (2nd. ed.). New York, NY: Oxford University Press.

Norcross, J. C. (2013). *Changeology: 5 steps to realizing your goals and resolutions*. New York, NY: Simon & Schuster.

Norcross, J. C., Beutler, L. E., & Levant, R. F. (Eds.). (2006a). *Evidence-based practices in mental health: Debate and dialogue on the fundamental questions*. Washington, DC: American Psychological Association.

Norcross, J. C., Campbell, L. M., Grohol, J. M., Santrock, J. W., Selagea, F., & Sommer, R. (2013). *Self-help that works: Resources to improve emotional health and strengthen relationships* (4th ed.). New York, NY: Oxford University Press.

Norcross, J. C., Koocher, G. P., Fala, N. C., & Wexler, H. K. (2010). What doesn't work? Expert consensus on discredited treatments in the addictions. *Journal of Addiction Medicine, 4*(3), 174–180. doi:10.1097/ADM.0b013e3181c5f9db

Norcross, J. C., Koocher, G. P., & Garofalo, A. (2006b). Discredited psychological treatments and tests: A Delphi poll. *Professional Psychology: Research & Practice, 37*, 515–522.

Norcross, J. C., Krebs, P. M., & Prochaska, J. O. (2011). Stages of change. In J. C. Norcross (Ed.), *Psychotherapy relationships that work* (2nd ed; pp. 279–300). New York, NY: Oxford University Press.

Norcross, J. C., & Lambert, M. J. (2006). The therapy relationship. In J. C. Norcross, L. E. Beutler, & R. F. Levant (Eds.), *Evidence-based practices in mental health: Debate and dialogue on the fundamental questions* (pp. 208–218). Washington, DC: American Psychological Association.

Osler, W. (1906). *Aequanimitas*. New York, NY: McGraw-Hill.

Oxford University Cochrane Library tutorial, learntech.physiol.ox.ac.uk/cochrane_tutorial/cochlibdoe4.php

Oxman, A. D., Thomson, M. A., Davis, D. A., & Haynes, R. B. (1995). No magic bullets: A systematic review of 102 trials of interventions to improve professional practice. *Canadian Medical Association Journal, 153*, 1423–1431.

Pagoto, S. L., Spring, B., Coups, E. J., Mulvaney, S., Coutu, M., & Ozakinci, G. (2007). Barriers and facilitators of evidence-based practice perceived by behavioral science health professionals. *Journal of Clinical Psychology, 63*, 695–705.

Parkes, J., Hyde, C., Deeks, J., & Milne, R. (2001). Teaching critical appraisal skills in health care setting. *Cochrane Database of Systematic Reviews* (3), CD001270. doi:10.1002/14651858. CD001270

Perkins, E. (2001). Johns Hopkins tragedy: Could librarians have prevented a death? newsbreaks.infotoday.com/nbreader.asp?Article ID=17534

Peterson, D. R. (1995). The reflective educator. *American Psychologist, 50,* 975–983.

Petitti, D. B. (2000). *Meta-analysis, decision analysis, and cost-effectiveness: Methods for quantitative synthesis in medicine* (2nd ed.). New York, NY: Oxford University Press.

President's New Freedom Commission on Mental Health. (2003). store.samhsa.gov/shin/content/SMA03-3831/SMA03-3831.pdf

Prochaska, J. O., DiClemente, C. C., & Norcross, J. C. (1992). In search of how people change: Applications to addictive behaviors. *American Psychologist, 47,* 1102–1114.

Prochaska, J. O., & Norcross, J. C. (2014). *Systems of psychotherapy: A transtheoretical analysis* (8th ed.). Stamford, CT: Cengage.

Prochaska, J. O., Norcross, J. C., & DiClemente, C. C. (1995). *Changing for good.* New York, NY: Avon.

Prochaska, J. O., Norcross, J. C., & DiClemente, C. C. (2005). Stages of change: Prescriptive guidelines. In G. P. Koocher, J. C. Norcross, & S. S. Hill (Eds.), *Psychologists' desk reference* (2nd ed.). New York, NY: Oxford University Press.

Rakovshik, S. G., McManus, F., Vazquez-Montes, M., Muse, K., & Ougrin, D. (2016). Is supervision necessary? Examining the effects of Internet-based CBT training with and without supervision. *Journal of Consulting and Clinical Psychology, 84*(3), 191–199. doi:10.1037/ccp0000079

Reavley, N. J., Mackinnon, A. J., Morgan, A. J., Alvarez-Jimenez, M., Hetrick, S. E., Killackey, E., . . . Jorm, A. F. (2012). Quality of information sources about mental disorders: A comparison of Wikipedia with centrally controlled Web and printed sources. *Psychological Medicine, 42,* 1753–1762.

Richardson, W. S., Wilson, M. C., Nishikawa, J., & Hayward, R. S. (1995). The well-built clinical question: A key to evidence-based decisions. *ACP Journal Club, 123*(3), A12–A13.

Rogers, E. M. (2003). *Diffusion of innovations* (5th ed.). New York, NY: Free Press.

Rosen, C. S. (2000). Is the sequencing of change processes by stage consistent across health problems? A meta-analysis. *Health Psychology, 19,* 593–604.

Rotheram-Borus, M. J., Swendeman, D., & Chorpita, B. F. (2012). Disruptive innovations for designing and diffusing evidence-based interventions. *American Psychologist, 67,* 463–476.

Royse, D., Thyer, B., & Padgett, D. (2015). *Program evaluation: An introduction to an evidence-based approach.* Belmont, CA: Cengage Learning.

Ruscio, A. M., & Holohan, D. R. (2006). Applying empirically supported treatments to complex cases: Ethical, empirical, and practical considerations. *Clinical Psychology: Science and Practice, 13,* 146–162.

Sackett, D. L., Straus, S. E., Richardson, W. S., Rosenberg, W., & Haynes, R. B. (2000). *Evidence-based medicine: How to practice and teach EBM* (2nd ed.). London: Churchill Livingstone.

Sagan, C. (1997). *The demon-haunted world: Science as a candle in the dark.* New York, NY: Random House.

SAMHSA Evidence-Based Practice Toolkits, store.samhsa.gov/list/series?name=Evidence-Based-Practices-KITs

Schardt, C., Adams, M. B., Owens, T., Keitz, J. A., & Fontelo, P. (2007). Utilization of the PICO framework to improve searching PubMed for clinical questions. *BMC Informatics and Decision Making, 7,* article 16.

Schilling, M. F., Watkins, A. E., & Watkins, W. (2002). Is human height bimodal? *The American Statistician, 56,* 223–229.

Schneider, M. S., Brown, L. S., & Glassgold, J. M. (2002). Implementing the Resolution on Appropriate Therapeutic Responses to Sexual Orientation: A guide for the perplexed. *Professional Psychology, 33,* 265–276.

Schulz, K.F., Altman, D. G., Moher, D., & CONSORT Group. (2010). CONSORT 2010 statement: Updated guidelines for reporting parallel group randomised trials. *Annals of Internal Medicine, 152*(11), 726–732. doi:10.7326/0003-4819-152-11-201006010-002322

Schumacker, R. E., & Lomax, R. G. (2016). *A beginner's guide to structural equation modeling* (4th ed). New York, NY: Routledge.

Searching for Evidence, www.ebbp.org/course_outlines/searching_for_evidence/

Semple, D., Smyth, R., Burns, J., Darjee, R., & McIntosh, A. (Eds.). (2005). *Oxford handbook of psychiatry.* New York, NY: Oxford University Press.

Shariff, S. Z., Bejaimal, S. A., Sontrop, J. M., Iansavichus, A. V., Haynes, R. B., Weir, M. A., & Garg, A. X. (2013). Retrieving clinical evidence: A comparison of PubMed and Google Scholar for quick clinical searches. *Journal of Medical Internet Research, 15*(8), e164.

Sheehan, A. K., Walrath, C. M., & Holden, E. W. (2007). Evidence-based practice use, training and implementation in the community-based service setting: A survey of children's mental health service providers. *Journal of Child and Family Studies, 16,* 169–183.

Smith, G. C. S., & Pell, J. P. (2003). Parachute use to prevent death and major trauma related to gravitational challenge: Systematic review of randomised controlled trials. *British Journal of Medicine, 327,* 1459. doi:dx.doi.org/10.1136/bmj.327.7429.1459

Smith, T. B., Rodriguez, M. D., & Bernal, G. (2011). Culture. In J. C. Norcross (Ed.), *Psychotherapy relationships that work* (2nd ed., pp. 316–335). New York, NY: Oxford University Press.

Spielmans, G. I., Gatlin, E. T., & McFall, J. P. (2010). The efficacy of evidence-based psychotherapies versus usual care for youths: Controlling confounds in a meta-reanalysis. *Psychotherapy Research, 20,* 234–246.

Spring, B., Pagoto, S., Knatterud, G., Kozak, A., & Hedeker, D. (2007). Examination of the analytic quality of behavioral health randomized clinical trials. *Journal of Clinical Psychology, 63,* 53–71.

Spring, B., & Walker, B. B. (Eds.). (2007). Evidence-based practice in clinical psychology: Education and training issues [Special issue]. *Journal of Clinical Psychology, 63*(7).

Stacey, D., Légaré, F., Col, N. F., Bennett, C. L., Barry, M. J., Eden, K. B., . . . Wu, J. H. C. (2014). Decision aids for people facing health treatment or screening decisions. *Cochrane Database of Systematic Reviews* (1), CD001431. doi:10.1002/14651858. CD001431.pub4

Stein, B. D., Celedonia, K. L., Swartz, H. A., DeRosier, M. E., Sorbero, M. J., Brindley, R. A., . . . Frank, E. (2015). Implementing a Web-based intervention to train community clinicians in an evidence-based psychotherapy: A pilot study. *Psychiatric Services, 66,* 988–991.

Stewart, R. E., & Chambless, D. L. (2009). Interesting practitioners in training in empirically supported treatments: Research reviews versus case studies. *Journal of Clinical Psychology, 66,* 73–95.

Stewart, R. E., & Chambless, D. L. (2010). What do clinicians want? An investigation of EST training desires. *The Clinical Psychologist, 63*(1), 5–10.

Stewart, R. E., Chambless, D. L., & Baron, J. (2011). Theoretical and practical barriers to practitioners' willingness to seek training and empirically supported treatments. *Journal of Clinical Psychology, 68*, 8–23.

Straus, S. E., Richardson, W. S., Glasziou, P., & Haynes, R. B. (2005). *Evidence-based medicine: How to practice and teach EBM* (3rd ed.). London, UK: Elsevier.

Straus, S. E., Richardson, W. S., Glasziou, P., & Haynes, R. B. (2010). *Evidence-based medicine: How to practice and teach EBM* (4th ed.). London, UK: Elsevier.

Strupp, H. H., & Hadley, S. W. (1977). A tripartite model of mental health and therapeutic outcomes. *American Psychologist, 32*, 187–194.

Sue, S., & Lam, A. G. (2002). Cultural and demographic diversity. In J. C. Norcross (Ed.), *Psychotherapy relationships that work: Therapist contributions and responsiveness to patients* (pp. 401–421). New York, NY: Oxford University Press.

Swift, J. K., Callahan, J. L., & Vollmer, B. M. (2011). Preferences. In J. C. Norcross (Ed.), *Psychotherapy relationships that work* (2nd ed., pp. 301–315). New York, NY: Oxford University Press.

Swift, J. K., & Greenberg, R. P. (2012). Premature discontinuation in adult psychotherapy: A meta-analysis. *Journal of Consulting and Clinical Psychology, 80*, 547–559. dx.doi.org/10.1037/a0028226

Tabachnick, B. G., & Fidell, L. S. (2013). *Using multivariate statistics* (6th ed.). Boston, MA: Pearson.

Tasca, G. A., Balfour, L., Evans, J., Francis, K., Huehn, L., Joyce, A. S., & Wilson, B. (2015). What clinicians want: Findings from a psychotherapy practice research network survey. *Psychotherapy, 52*, 1–11.

Tashiro, T., & Mortensen, L. (2006). Translational research: How social psychology can improve psychotherapy. *American Psychologist, 61*, 959–966.

Thyer, B. A., & Wodarski, J. S. (Eds.). (2007). *Social work in mental health: An evidence-based approach.* New York, NY: Wiley.

Tryon, G. S., Collins, S., & Felleman, E. (2006, August). *Meta-analysis of the third session client–therapist working alliance.*

Paper presented at the annual convention of the American Psychological Association, New Orleans, LA.

Tryon, G. S., & Winograd, G. (2011). Goal consensus and collaboration. In J. C. Norcross (Ed.), *Psychotherapy relationships that work* (2nd ed., pp. 109–125). New York, NY: Oxford University Press.

Tukey, J. W. (1977). *Exploratory data analysis.* Reading, MA: Addison-Wesley.

Tuleya, L. G. (2007). *Thesaurus of psychological index terms.* Washington, DC: American Psychological Association.

Turk, D. C., & Salovey, P. (Eds.). (1988). *Reasoning, inference, and judgment in clinical psychology.* New York, NY: Free Press.

Types of Clinical Questions, guides.dml.georgetown.edu/ebm/ebmclinicalquestions

Ullman, J. B. (2012). Structural equation modeling. In B. G. Tabachnick & L. S. Fidell, *Using multivariate statistics* (6th ed., pp. 681–785). Boston, MA: Allyn and Bacon.

van Assen, M. A. L. M., van Aert, R. C. M., & Wicherts, J. M. (2015). Meta-analysis using effect size distributions of only statistically significant studies. *Psychological Methods, 20,* 293–309.

Vandewaetere, M., Manhaeve, D., Aertgeerts, B., Clarebout, G., Van Merriënboer, J. J., & Roex, A. (2015). 4C/ID in medical education: How to design an educational program based on whole-task learning: AMEE Guide No. 93. *Medical Teacher, 37,* 4–20.

van Merrienboer, J. J. G. (1997). *Training complex cognitive skills: A four-component instructional design model.* Englewood Cliffs, NJ: Educational Technology.

Villanueva, E. V., Burrows, E. A., Fennessy, P. A., Rajendran, M., & Anderson, J. N. (2001). Improving question formulation in evidence appraisal in a tertiary care setting: A randomized controlled trial. *BMC Informatics and Decision Making, 1,* article 4.

Walker, B. B., Seay, S. J., Solomon, A. C., & Spring, B. (2006). Treating chronic migraine headaches: An evidence-based practice approach. *Journal of Clinical Psychology: In Session, 62,* 1367–1378.

Wallerstein, R. S. (1986). *Forty-two lives in treatment.* New York, NY: Guilford.

Wampold, B. E., & Bhati, K. S. (2004). Attending to the omissions: A historical examination of evidence-based practice movements. *Professional Psychology: Research and Practice, 35,* 563–570.

Wampold, B. E., & Imel, Z. E. (2015). *The great psychotherapy debate: The evidence for what makes psychotherapy work* (2nd ed.). New York, NY: Routledge.

Waserstein, R. L., & Lazar, N. A. (2016). The ASA's statement on p-values: Context, process, and purpose. *The American Statistician, 70*(2), 129–133. doi:10.1080/00031305.2016.1154108

Webb, C. A., DeRubeis, R. J., & Barber, J. P. (2010). Therapist adherence/competence and treatment outcome: A meta-analytic review. *Journal of Consulting and Clinical Psychology, 78,* 200–211. dx.doi.org/10.1037/a0018912

Weisz, J. R., Jensen-Doss, A., & Hawley, K. M. (2006). Evidence-based youth psychotherapies versus usual clinical care. *American Psychologist, 61,* 671–689.

Westen, D. I. (2006). Patients and treatments in clinical trials are not adequately representative of clinical practice. In J. C. Norcross, L. E. Beutler, & R. F. Levant (Eds.), *Evidence-based practices in mental health: Debate and dialogue on the fundamental questions* (pp. 161–171). Washington, DC: American Psychological Association.

Westen, D., & Morrison, K. (2001). A multidimensional meta-analysis of treatments for depression, panic, and generalized anxiety disorder: An empirical examination of the status of empirically supported therapies. *Journal of Consulting and Clinical Psychology, 69,* 875–899.

Westen, D., Novotny, C., & Thompson-Brenner, H. (2004). The empirical status of empirically supported therapies: Assumptions, methods, and findings. *Psychological Bulletin, 130,* 631–663.

Whaley, A. L., & Davis, K. E. (2007). Cultural competence and evidence-based practice in mental health services. *American Psychologist, 62,* 563–574.

Wilkinson, L., & APA Task Force on Statistical Inference. (1999). Statistical methods in psychology journals: Guidelines and explanations. *American Psychologist, 54,* 594–604.

Wilson, G. T. (1995). Empirically validated treatments as a basis for clinical practice: Problems and prospects. In S. C. Hayes, V. M. Follette, R. M. Dawes, & K. E. Grady (Eds.), *Scientific standards of psychological practice* (pp. 163–196). Reno, NV: Context Press.

Wilson, J. L., Armoutliev, E., Yakunina, E., & Werth, J. L. (2009). Practicing psychologists' reflections on evidence-based practice in psychology. *Professional Psychology: Research and Practice, 40,* 403–409.

Witkiewitz, K. A., & Marlatt, G. A. (Eds.). (2007). *Therapist's guide to evidence-based relapse prevention.* London, UK: Elsevier.

Woody, R. H. (2013). Defending against legal (malpractice and licensing) complaints. In G. P. Koocher, J. C. Norcross, & B. A. Greene (Eds.), *Psychologists' desk reference* (3rd ed.). New York, NY: Oxford University Press.

World Health Organization (2011). *Mental health atlas 2011.* Geneva, Switzerland: Author.

Worthington, E. L., Jr., Hook, J. N., Davis, D. E., & McDaniel, M. A. (2011). Religion and spirituality. In J. C. Norcross (Ed.), *Psychotherapy relationships that work* (2nd ed., pp. 402–420). New York, NY: Oxford University Press.

Wu, Y. P., Aylward, B. S., Roberts, M. C., & Evans, S. C. (2012). Searching the scientific literature: Implications for quantitative and qualitative reviews. *Clinical Psychology Review, 32,* 553–557.

Wyer, P. C., Keitz, S., Hatala, R., Hayward, R., Barratt, A., Montori, V., . . . Guyatt, G. (2004). Tips for learning and teaching evidence-based medicine: Introduction to the series. *Canadian Medical Journal Association, 171,* 77–81.

Youngstrom, E. A., Choukas-Bradley, S., Calhoun, C. D., & Jensen-Doss, A. (2015). Clinical guide to the evidence-based assessment approach to diagnosis and treatment. *Cognitive and Behavioral Practice, 22*(1), 20–35.

Zwi, M., Jones, H., Thorgaard, C., York, A., & Dennis, J.A. (2011). Parent training interventions for attention deficit hyperactivity disorder (ADHD) in children aged 5 to 18 years. *Cochrane Database of Systematic Reviews* (12), CD003018. doi:10.1002/14651858.CD003018.pub3

Index

References to figures, tables and boxes are denoted by an italicized *f*, *t*, and *b*.

4C/ID (Four Component Instruction Design), 259–60, 261*t*
AAA TIE (triple A TIE), 14, 160
definition, 269, 273
evaluation in, 219
part-task practice, 260, 261*t*
teaching and supervision, 259
Aarons, Gregory, 250
Access Medicine, 35
actuarial judgment, 225, 269
Addiction Technology Transfer Center Network, 37
adopt it, adapt it, or abandon it, 211, 269
adults, discredited mental health treatments, 178*b*
Advances in Psychotherapy: Evidence-Based Practice (series), 35
advertising, 244–45
albuterol, 13, 183, 184*f*, 241
Alcoholics Anonymous, 1, 20
alcoholism, 20
alpha level (α), 72, 269, 281, 283
American Academy of Child and Adolescent Psychiatry, 41
American Academy of Pediatrics, 230
American Journal of Psychiatry (journal), 47
American Psychological Association (APA), 2–3, 280
ethics code, 239, 240*t*
analysis of covariance (ANCOVA), 89, 269–70
analysis of variance (ANOVA), 79, 270
anchoring effect, 222*t*
Annique (patient), 14
arbitrary metrics, 228
health insurance, 175
integrating components of EBP, 200–205
questions, 19
risk-taking, 234
self-report, 228
treatment research, 66–67
APA Task Force on Evidence-Based Practice, 4, 5, 166

appraisal of research reports. *See* research report appraisal
arbitrary metrics, 228, 270
audience, *xvi*
audit, 226, 231–32, 270
authority-based practice, 2, 270
availability bias, 222*t*

background information, 30–31
background information resources, 34–41, 41*b*
eMedicine, 36–37
practice guidelines, 40–41
textbooks, 34–36
UpToDate, 36
websites, 37–40
background questions, 19–20, 270, 276
Barnum effect, 222*t*
base rate, 124, 270, 280
base rate neglect, 222*t*
Beck Depression Inventory (BDI), 64, 115
behavioral health and addictions
myths about EBPs in, 257*b*
psychosocial model, 192–93
benchmarks, 226, 270
comparing patient outcomes, 230–31
effect size, 119, 275
best available research, 5, 270–71
background information, 30–31
background information resources, 34–41
filtered information, 31
ideal *vs.* typical search process, 30
see also research
bias, 172–74
bivariate outlier, 133
blended learning, 253, 271
BMJ Clinical Evidence, 42, 45–46, 271
Bonferroni correction, 75, 271
Boolean operators, 32–33, 271
Buros, Oscar, 65
Buros website, 65, 66–67, 271

Campbell Collaboration (C₂), 42, 44, 118, 271
Campbell Collaboration Reviews of Interventions and Policy Evaluations, 44, 271
case study method, 93, 271
causal modeling, 100
causal words, 90
CDSR (Cochrane Database of Systematic Reviews), 42–44, 59, 272
CENTRAL (Cochrane Central Register of Controlled Trials), 59, 61b
Centre for Evidence-Based Mental Health, 257
children, discredited mental health treatments, 178b
CINAHL (Cumulative Index to Nursing and Allied Health Literature), 2, 3f, 54–55, 61b, 271
clinical decision making
  adopt, adapt or abandon, 211–16, 269
  analysis, 182–87
  clinical expertise and, 193–95
  in complex cases, 205–6, 209–11
  decision aids, 198
  evidence-based practice and, 192–93
  integrating components of EBP, 199–205
  patient characteristics, cultures and preferences, 193, 195–99
  psychosocial model and, 192–93
clinical expertise, 5–6, 193–95, 272
clinical practice application
  assessing potential harm, 174–76
  becoming reflective practitioners, 165–66
  decision analysis, 182–87
  identifying discredited practices, 176–77, 178–79b
  randomized clinical trials (RCTs), 166–72
  translational research, 164–65, 247–48
clinical questions, 17–26
  asking patients, 25–26
  background, 19–20
  foreground, 20
  PICO format, 21–24
  prioritization, 26
  unanswerable, 18–19
  usefulness of, 17–18
Clinical Trials Network (CTN), 264
cluster samples, 150
Cochrane, Archie, 2
Cochrane Central Register of Controlled Trials (CENTRAL), 59, 61b
Cochrane Collaboration, 2, 147
Cochrane Database of Systematic Reviews (CDSR), 42–44, 59, 272
Cochrane Library, 272
Cochrane Review, 29–30

cocreation, 262, 272
Cohen's d, 117, 119f, 120f, 139, 272
cohort, 206, 272
comorbid disorders, 206, 207b, 209, 272
companion website, xix, 267
comparison, PICO format, 21–24
comparison group, research studies, 155–56, 160
competence, ethics, 239, 241–42
complex cases
  common features of, 207–8b
  integrating components of EBP, 205–6, 209–11
Comprehensive Meta-Analysis, software, 147
conclusions vs. actual results, research studies, 156–57, 160
confidence-based practice, 12
confidence interval (CI), 73, 111, 272, 279, 282
  odds ratio (OR), 127
  reliability of, 114
  for statistics, 114–16
  for test score, 111–14
confirmation bias, 222t, 224
confirmatory factor analysis (CFA), 98–99, 101, 272
confound, 88, 273
conjunction fallacy, 222t
consent, 242–43
CONSORT (Consolidated Standards of Reporting Trials), 151, 158, 163, 180
  checklist for reporting randomized trial, 169–70, 173
  flow chart, 151f, 168
controlled vocabularies, 50–51, 273
convenience samples, 149, 273
core EBP skills, 14, 273
Cork Database, 59–60, 61b
corrections for attenuation, 141, 273
cost-benefit analysis, 175, 273
criterion problem, 228–29, 273
critical appraisal, 137, 148–60, 273
critical incident stress debriefing (CISD), 177
CTN (Clinical Trials Network), 264
cultural adaptation, 214–15, 273
Cumulative Index to Nursing and Allied Health Literature (CINAHL), 2, 3f, 54–55, 61b, 271
cut score, 129, 274, 278, 280

damages, 236
Database of Abstracts of Reviews of Effects (DARE), 42, 45
databases, 2, 3
  test information, 64–65

Daubert v. Merrell Dow Pharmaceuticals, Inc. (1993), 172, 236–38
decision aids, 198, 274
decision analysis, 175, 182–87, 274
departure from standard of care, 235, 274
dependent variable, 82, 154–55, 159, 274
dereliction, 235
Diagnostic and Statistical Manual of Mental Disorders (DSM–IV), 210
Diagnostic Interview Schedule for Children (DISC), 185
direct causation, 235
discredited practices, 176–77, 178–79b, 274
dissemination, 251–52, 274, 277, 282
double-blind design, 156
duty, 235

EBSCO, library vendor, 55, 56, 57, 66
effectiveness, evaluation of
    practitioner performance, 221–31
    profession, 232–33
    program or organization, 231–32
    risk management and, 233–39
effectiveness research, 165–66, 275
effect size benchmarks, 119, 275
effect size (ES), 73, 116–23, 274
    benchmarks, 119, 275
    common measures of, 117–18
    frameworks for interpreting, 121t
    graphic illustrations of, 119–20
    measures of, 73, 119, 121–22
    meta-analysis, 139
    other descriptors of, 120–21
    proportion of variance in common, 122–23
efficacy research, 165–66, 275
eMedicine Clinical Knowledge Database, 36–37, 274
eminence-based practice, 11
epidemiology, 184, 275
error score, 111–12, 275
e-texts, 34–35, 41b, 63
ethics
    advertising, 244–45
    competence, 239, 241–42
    consent, 242–43
    public statements, 244–45
    relationship of EBP to principles, 240t
ETS (Educational Testing Service) Test Collection, 64–65, 67, 275
evaluation. *See* effectiveness, evaluation of
Evidence-Based Behavioral Practice, 256–57
evidence-based journals, 46–47
evidence-based medicine (EBM), 2, 5, 275
Evidence-Based Mental Health (journal), 46–47

Evidence-Based Practice Attitude Scale (EBPAS), 250
evidence-based practice (EBP), *xv*, 1
    4C/ID model (Four Component Instruction Design), 259–60, 261t
    alternatives to, 11–12
    audience, *xvi*
    barriers to adoption and implementation of, 250–51
    clients, *xvii*
    clinical decision making and, 192–93
    conceptual framework of, 253–55
    controversies, 7–11
    core skills, 14, 255–59
    definition of, 4–6, 275
    disseminating, 251–52
    ethics, *xviii*
    ethics and, 239–45
    goal of, *xvi–xvii*, 6–7
    implementation of, 262–65
    integrating three components of, 199–205
    mnemonics, 259
    myths about behavioral health and addictions, 257b
    patients, 13–14
    pernicious myths about, 190–92
    pillars of, 189–90
    practitioners drawn to, 248–50
    search engines, 61–63
    short history of, 1–4
stages of change in adoption of, 220t
    teaching, 252–62
exploratory factor analysis (EFA), 98

factor analysis, 97–99, 275
factorial designs, 85–87
false consensus bias, 222t
false negatives, 131–32, 275
false positives, 131–32, 276
fidelity, 212, 263, 276
filtered information sources, 30, 31, 276
    BMJ Clinical Evidence, 42, 45–46
    Campbell Collaboration (C₂), 42, 44
    Cochrane Database of Systematic Reviews (CDSR), 42–44
    Database of Abstracts of Reviews of Effects (DARE), 42, 45
    evidence-based journals, 46–47
    resources, 42–47
five A's, 259, 276
foreground questions, 20, 270, 276
forest plot, meta-analysis, 142–44
fortune teller effect, 222t
Four Component Instruction Design (4C/ID), 259–60, 261t
four Ds of legal liability, 235–36, 276

framing effect, 222*t*
Francesco (patient), 13
    arbitrary metrics, 228
    generalized anxiety disorder (GAD), 154
    lacking health insurance, 176
    PICO strategy, 22
    questions, 19
    risk-taking, 234
    self-report, 227
Freud, Sigmund, 7, 93
Frye standard, 237
F-test, 79–80
funnel plot, meta-analysis, 145–46
fuzzy definition of independent variable, 152

gambler's fallacy, 222*t*
generalizability theory, 114
generalization, 258, 276
generalized anxiety disorder (GAD), 13
gold standard, 82–84
Goodman and Gilman's The Pharmacological
    Basis of Therapeutics (Knollmann), 35,
    41*b*
Google, 29, 39, 40, 41*b*
Google Scholar, 39, 60–61, 61*b*, 276
Great Expectations (Dickens), 12
gross negligence, 235, 276
groupthink, 223*t*

Health and Psychosocial Instruments (HaPI)
    database, 64
Health Care Innovations Exchange, 4
health professions, evaluation of, 232–33
Hedge's formula, 117
heuristic biases, 222–23*t*
heuristics, 221, 276
hits, 132, 277
homogeneity bias, 223*t*, 224
hypotheses, 69–80
    null hypothesis significance tests
        (NHSTs), 70–72
    objections to NHSTs, 72–73
    power and factors affecting, 76–78
    test statistics in NHST, 79–80
    types of errors in hypothesis testing, 73–76

implementation, 251, 274, 277
    barriers to, of EBPs, 250–51
    evidence-based practices, 262–65
implementation science, 262, 277, 282
independent variable, 81, 152–53, 159, 277
indexes of heterogeneity, meta-analysis,
    144–45
information
    expert assistance, 67–68
    tests and measures, 63–67
innovation, liability and, 236–39

Institute of Medicine (IOM), 4
intent-to-treat (ITT) analysis, 152
interaction, 85, 86*f*, 277
internal consistency reliability, 114
internal validity, 82
interpersonal psychotherapy (IPT), 200
interquartile range, 133
intervention, PICO format, 21–24
intervention effectiveness, 181*t*

Jonathan (patient), 13
    albuterol, 13, 183, 184*f*, 241
    arbitrary metrics, 228
    confidence intervals (CIs), 113
    decision tree for diagnosis of, 184*f*
    decision tree for treatment of, 186*f*
    family and individual therapy, 43
    integrating components of EBP, 203–4
    PICO strategy, 22
    questions, 19
journals, evidence-based, 46–47
junk science, 238

Kraepelin, Emil, 1
Kumho Tire Co., Ltd. v. Carmichael (1999),
    238
kurtosis, 110

Lake Wobegon effect, 223*t*
latent variables, 101
LexisNexis, 58–59, 61*b*
liability, 236–39
lifetime prevalence rate, 124
literature research
    Cochrane Central Register of Controlled
        Trials (CENTRAL), 59
    controlled vocabularies, 50–51
    Cork Database, 59–60
    Cumulative Index to Nursing and Allied
        Health Literature (CINAHL), 54–55
    evidence-based practice search engines,
        61–63
    expert assistance, 67–68
    Google Scholar, 60–61
    LexisNexis, 58–59
    MEDLINE, 51–53
    PsycINFO, 56–57
    PubMed clinical queries, 54
    Social Services Abstracts, 55–56
    tests and measures, 63–67
    unfiltered sources, 49–68
logistic regression, 96–97, 277

McMaster University Group, 2
main effect, 85, 277
maintenance, 258, 277
margin of error, 91

measures. *See* numbers and measures; tests and measures
mediation analysis, 103–5
mediator, 103–5, 153, 277
Medical Subject Headings (MeSH), 50–51, 277
MEDLINE, 2, 3*f*, 51–53, 61*b*, 277, 281
mental health treatments, discredited practices, 178*b*
Mental Measurements Yearbook (MMY), 65–66, 278
meta-analysis, 139–41, 278
  advanced techniques for, 141–42
  checklist of, 148
  forest plot, 142–44
  funnel plot, 145–46
  indexes of heterogeneity, 144–45
  meta-regression, 145
  methods for reporting, 142–48
  moderator analyses, 145
  publication bias, 146–47
  software for, 147–48
meta-regression, meta-analysis, 145
The Mill on the Floss (Eliot), 190
misperceptions of randomness, 223*t*
modality, 110
moderator, 153, 278
moderator analyses, meta-analysis, 145
multiple correlation, 95
multiple regression, 95–96, 277, 278
multivariate analysis of variance (MANOVA), 79
multivariate techniques, 93–106
  confirmatory factor analysis (CFA), 98–99, 101
  factor analysis, 97–99
  logistic regression, 96–97
  mediation analysis, 103–5
  multiple regression, 95–96
  partial correlation, 93–95
  structural equation modeling (SEM), 99–103

narrative review, 139, 278
National Association of Social Workers, 55
National Child Traumatic Stress Network, 38–39
National Guideline Clearinghouse, 3, 41
National Implementation Research Network (NIRN), 251
National Institute for Health and Clinical Excellence (NICE), 41
National Institute of Drug Abuse (NIDA), 264
National Institute of Mental Health (NIMH), 125, 149, 164
National Library of Medicine, 35, 41*b*, 277

National Registry of Evidence-Based Programs and Practices (NREPP), 37–38, 41*b*, 278
natural group contrasts, 87–88
natural language, 21, 278
negative predictive power (NPP), 130–31, 278
negative skewness, 111
nervousness-based practice, 11
New England Journal of Medicine (journal), 62
New Freedom Commission on Mental Health, 11
NICE (National Institute for Health and Clinical Excellence), 41
NIDA (National Institute of Drug Abuse), 264
NIMH (National Institute of Mental Health), 125, 149, 164
NIRN (National Implementation Research Network), 251
normal curve, 109–11
"not my fault" bias, 223*t*, 224
NREPP (National Registry of Evidence-Based Programs and Practices), 37–38, 41*b*, 278
null hypothesis, 69–70, 278, 281
null hypothesis significance test (NHST), 70–72, 278
  objections to, 72–73
  standard error of a statistic, 71–72
  types of error in, 73–76
numbers and measures, 109–34
  checklist for, 133–34
  confidence intervals and standard errors, 111–16
  effect size, 116–23
  false positives and false negatives, 131–32
  normal curve, 109–11
  odds ratio, 125–27, 128
  outliers, 132–33
  relative rates and related ratios, 124–25
  relative risk, 127, 128
  selectivity, specificity and predictive power, 128–31

observational studies, 92–93
obtained score, 111–12, 278
odds ratio (OR), 97, 125–27, 128, 278
opportunistic bias, 173, 279
OR confidence interval, 279
Osler, Sir William, 205
Outcome, PICO format, 21–24
outlier, 132–33, 279
Oxford Clinical Psychology, 36, 41*b*

paradoxical interventions, 210, 279
parameter, 114, 279, 282

parent management training, 214–15
partial correlation, 93–95, 279
path model, 100*f*
patient, PICO format, 21–24
patient characteristics, culture and
    preferences, 6, 193, 195–99, 279
patient diversity, 10
patient outcomes
    comparing with benchmarks, 230–31
    tracking, 226–30
patient preferences, 25, 213, 279
pattern, 133
pay for performance (P_4P), 233, 279
PICO (patient, intervention, comparison,
    outcome), 20
    format, 29, 279
    questions, 21–24, 53
PICOT (patient, intervention, comparison,
    outcome, and type of question), 20, 22
placebo, 155–56, 280
point biserial correlation, 122
positive predictive power (PPP), 130–31, 280
positive skewness, 111
potential harm, assessment of, 174–76
power, 76–78, 280
practice-based evidence, 12, 280
practice guidelines, 40–41, 226, 230, 280
practitioner performance evaluation, 221–31
    audit of work, 226, 231–32
    benchmark comparisons, 230–31
    heuristic biases, 222–23*t*
    practice guidelines, 230
    tracking patient outcomes, 226–30
practitioners
    determining bias, 172–74
    propensity to use EBPs, 248–50
    reflective, 165–66, 216–17
predict, 90
predictive power, 128–31
preferences, 25, 213, 279
prevalence rate, 124–25, 270, 280
proportion of variance in common, 122–23,
    280
providence-based practice, 11
proxy consent, 243
psychological tests, discredited practices,
    179*b*
psychosocial model, behavioral health and
    addiction, 192–93
Psychotherapy (journal), 227
PsycINFO, 2, 3*f*, 30, 49, 56–57, 61*b*, 280
PsycTESTS, 65, 280
publication, 9–10
publication bias, 146–47, 280–81
Publication Manual of the American
    Psychological Association, 73

public statements, 244–45
publishers, tests, 66
PubMed, 30, 49, 51–53, 61*b*, 277, 281
PubMed Clinical Queries, 54, 61*b*

quasi-experimental designs, 87–89
    analysis of covariance (ANCOVA), 89
    natural group contrasts, 87–88
    time series designs, 88–89

random, 81, 281
random assignment, 84
randomized clinical trials (RCTs), 8, 42, 80–84,
    149, 163, 281
    CONSORT 2010 checklist for reporting,
        169–70*t*
    evaluating, 166–72
random sampling, 84
range restriction, 141, 281
reflective practitioner, 165–66, 216–17
relative risk, 127, 128, 281
reliability, 154
reparative therapies, 177
representativeness bias, 223*t*
research
    efficacy *vs.* effectiveness, 165–66
    inconsistent evidence, 180–82
    translational, 164–65, 247–48
    see also best available research
research designs
    case studies, 93
    factorial designs, 85–87
    identifying causal words, 90
    observational studies, 92–93
    quasi-experimental designs, 87–89
    survey designs, 90–92
    true experimental design, 80–84
research hypothesis, 69, 278, 281
research report appraisal
    checklist for, 148, 159–60
    comparison group characteristics, 155–56,
        160
    conclusions *vs.* actual results, 156–57, 160
    consequences of methodological
        malpractice, 157–58
    critical, 148–60
    dependent variable, 154–55, 159
    independent variable, 152–53, 159
    individual articles, 137–38
    meta-analyses, 139–42
    methods for reporting meta-analysis,
        142–48
    narrative reviews, 139
    sample characteristics and, 149–52, 159
Revised Hamilton Rating Scale for
    Depression (RHRSD), 66–67

RevMan, software, 147
right to refuse treatment, 243
risk-benefit analysis, 175, 216, 281
risk difference, 127, 128
risk management, 281
    evidence-based practices, 233–39
    liability and innovation, 236–39
    mistakes *vs.* negligence, 235–36
risk ratio, 127, 128
Rush, Benjamin, 1

SAMHSA (Substance Abuse and Mental
    Health Services Administration), 3, 37,
    41, 41*b*
sample, research studies, 149–52, 159
sampling distribution, 72
sampling frame, 91
scientific hypothesis, 69
search concepts, 32–34
    Boolean operators, 32–33
    truncation, 34
    Venn diagram of AND, 32*f*
    Venn diagram of OR, 33*f*
    wild cards, 33–34
search engines, evidence-based practice, 61–63
search process, ideal *vs.* typical, 30
selectivity, 281
self-confidence models, 101, 102*f*, 103
sensitivity, 128–31, 281
sexual orientation conversion, 177
sham placebo, 156
significance effect, publication bias, 147
significance level, 72, 281
significance test, 82, 281, 282
simple random sample, 150, 282
Single Citation Matcher, 53
Social Services Abstracts, 55–56, 61*b*
Society of Clinical Psychology, 38
specificity, 128–31, 282
standard error, confidence interval and, 111–16
standard error of measurement (SEM), 112,
    282
standard error of statistic, 71–72, 115, 282
standardized mean difference, 118, 282
standard of care, 233, 282
statistic, 114, 279, 282
statistical hypothesis, 69–70, 282
statistical software packages, 147–48
statistics, confidence intervals for, 114–16
stratified sample, 150
structural equation modeling (SEM), 99–103
Substance Abuse and Mental Health
    Services Administration (SAMHSA), 3,
    37, 41, 41*b*
substance abuse treatments, discredited
    practices, 179b

survey designs, 90–92
sustainability, 264, 282
symmetry, 110
systematic review, 139

talk page, Wikipedia, 39–40
target group, 128
teaching EBPs, 252–62
    4C/ID model (Four Component
        Instruction Design), 259–60, 261*t*
    clinician preferences, 260–62
    conceptual framework, 253–55
    core skills, 255–59
    mnemonics, 259
test-retest reliability, 114
tests and measures
    assessing information on, 63–67
    publishers of, 66
    reviews of, 65–66
    test information databases, 64–65
test score, confidence intervals for, 111–14
Tests in Print (TIP), 64
textbooks, 34–36
time series designs, 88–89
transdiagnostic, 210, 212, 215, 282
translational research, 164–65, 247–48, 282
transportability, 10, 166, 282
treatment, right to refuse, 243
treatment as usual (TAU), 156, 158, 173–74,
    283
Treatment of Adolescent Depression Study
    (TADS), 149
treatment outcomes, 8–9
Treatments That Work (Oxford paperbacks),
    35, 41*b*
triple A TIE. *See* AAA TIE (triple A TIE)
TRIP (Turning Research Into Practice)
    database, 62–63, 283
true experimental design, 80–84, 281, 283
true negatives, 132
true positives, 132
true score, 111–12, 283
truncation, 34, 283
truthiness, 223*t*
t-test, 79–80
Turning Research Into Practice (TRIP)
    database, 62–63, 283
Type I error, 73–75, 283
Type II error, 73, 74*f*, 76, 77, 280, 283

unfiltered information sources, 283
unimodal, normal curve, 110
univariate outlier, 133
UpToDate, 36, 41*b*, 283
US Centers for Disease Control and
    Prevention (CDC), 125

validation, 9, 10
validity, 154
vehemence-based practice, 11
Venn diagram, 216
    conceptual relationship of AND, 32*f*
    conceptual relationship
        of OR, 33*f*
    integrating components of EBP, 200*f*,
        201*f*, 203*f*, 204*f*

WebMD, 36–37

websites
    background information, 37–40
    companion for book, *xix*, 267
Wechsler Intelligence Scale for Children, 5th
    edition (WISC-V), 113
Wikipedia, 39–40, 41*b*
wild cards, 33–34, 283
World Health Organization
    (WHO), 125
wow effect, 223*t*, 224
Wundt, Wilhelm, 1

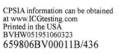

CPSIA information can be obtained
at www.ICGtesting.com
Printed in the USA
BVHW051951060323
659806BV00011B/436